CW01475934

INT

Anabolic
Edge

Secrets
For That
Extra Lean
Muscle Mass

By Phil Embleton
& Gerard Thorne

Copyright 1999 by Robert Kennedy

All rights reserved including the right to
reproduce this book or portions thereof
in any form whatsoever.

Published by MuscleMag International
6465 Airport Road
Mississauga, ON
Canada L4V 1E4

Designed by Jackie Kydyk

10 9 8 7 6 5 4 3 2 1 Pbk

Canadian Cataloguing in Publication Data

Embleton, Phil, 1963-
    Musclemag International's anabolic edge:
secrets for that extra lean muscle mass

Includes index.

ISBN 1-55210-016-2

    1. Bodybuilding--Physiological aspects.
2. Bodybuilders--Drug use. I. Thorne, Gerard, 1963-.
I. Title.

RC1220.W44E418 2000   613.7'11   C00-900003-8

Distributed in Canada by
CANBOOK Distribution Services
1220 Nicholson Road
Newmarket, ON
L3Y 7V1
800-399-6858

Distributed in the States by
BookWorld Services
1933 Whitfield Park Loop
Sarasota, FL 34243
800-444-2524

Printed in Canada

Anabolic Edge

Secrets For That Extra Lean Muscle Mass

ACKNOWLEDGMENTS

As with our previous works, the authors would like to thank a number of individuals for their assistance in writing this book.

To Mike Peddle and Carl Horwood, our sincere thanks for your computer expertise. After finally breaking down and going kicking and screaming into the computer age, it's nice to have such support behind you.

Our thanks to Karen Cross for tracking down many of the references used throughout this book. All the best in med school Karen!

To Jackie Kydyk and staff at *MuscleMag International*, thanks once again for giving our words such great visual appeal.

Finally, to Robert Kennedy, for giving us yet another opportunity to expand *MuscleMag International's* growing library of publications. We are happy to be able to contribute in our own small way.

Gerard Thorne and Phil Embleton

Table of Contents

Foreword

By Robert Kennedy

"It doesn't matter what anyone tells you, just do whatever you damn-well please!"

– My mother, on more than one occasion. In fact, almost daily during my fun-filled frolic through puberty.

"The only friend you've got is a buck! And the more bucks you've got, the more friends you've got!"

– Fred Flinstone, sharing his philosophy of life with side-kick, Barney Rubble.

Lately, I have been the subject of attack from a number of groups and individuals, both in print and on the internet. It is an unfortunate fact of life that the more success you enjoy, the more criticism you will draw. Isn't it amazing how someone can tell you you're doing something wrong, when what you're doing works?

I'm a prisoner of my time. The world of bodybuilding has grown, diversified and evolved at a dizzying pace. *MuscleMag International* continues to reach out to all members of our community, but the recent schism between natural (i.e. no anabolic steroids) and traditional (bring on the juice!) has erupted into a no-holds barred contest. Now when my staff puts a magazine together, we have to consider the balance of articles between the two groups in order to please our customers and our advertisers. Occasionally, a good story is dropped because it is just too controversial (this is daily reality at all major newspapers and news shows, just ask any journalist). Please understand, I'm not interested in being politically-correct (I'm not even sure what politically-correct is anymore). I'm more interested in the growth of my magazine, educating the bodybuilding public and paying my staff! As long as you, the reader, is happy with our product, then this will continue.

You see, in this business you're only as good as your last issue (in our case, that's reassuring). My point is, you can't please all of the people all of the time, so you may as well please yourself. Hardcore bodybuilders (lift heavy, eat huge, train hard, take weapons of mass construction) are one group that have been particularly displaced by recent events. They have genuine bitterness about this, because they were among the originators of modern bodybuilding, and responsible for much of the success of many publications, including *MuscleMag International*. This book, a complementary volume to the *Anabolic Primer*, is our attempt to reach out to them. This book is as hardcore as I can get without being imprisoned. Almost every pharmaceutical advantage that exists has been tracked down for your edification. Steroids and cycles, anticatabolic supplements and associated substances fill this book. My advice is to obey the law in your country, use common sense, eat wholesome natural foods for optimum health, don't do drugs, watch your cholesterol levels and pick up the latest issue of *MuscleMag International*. All the best.

Robert Kennedy,
Publisher of *MuscleMag International*

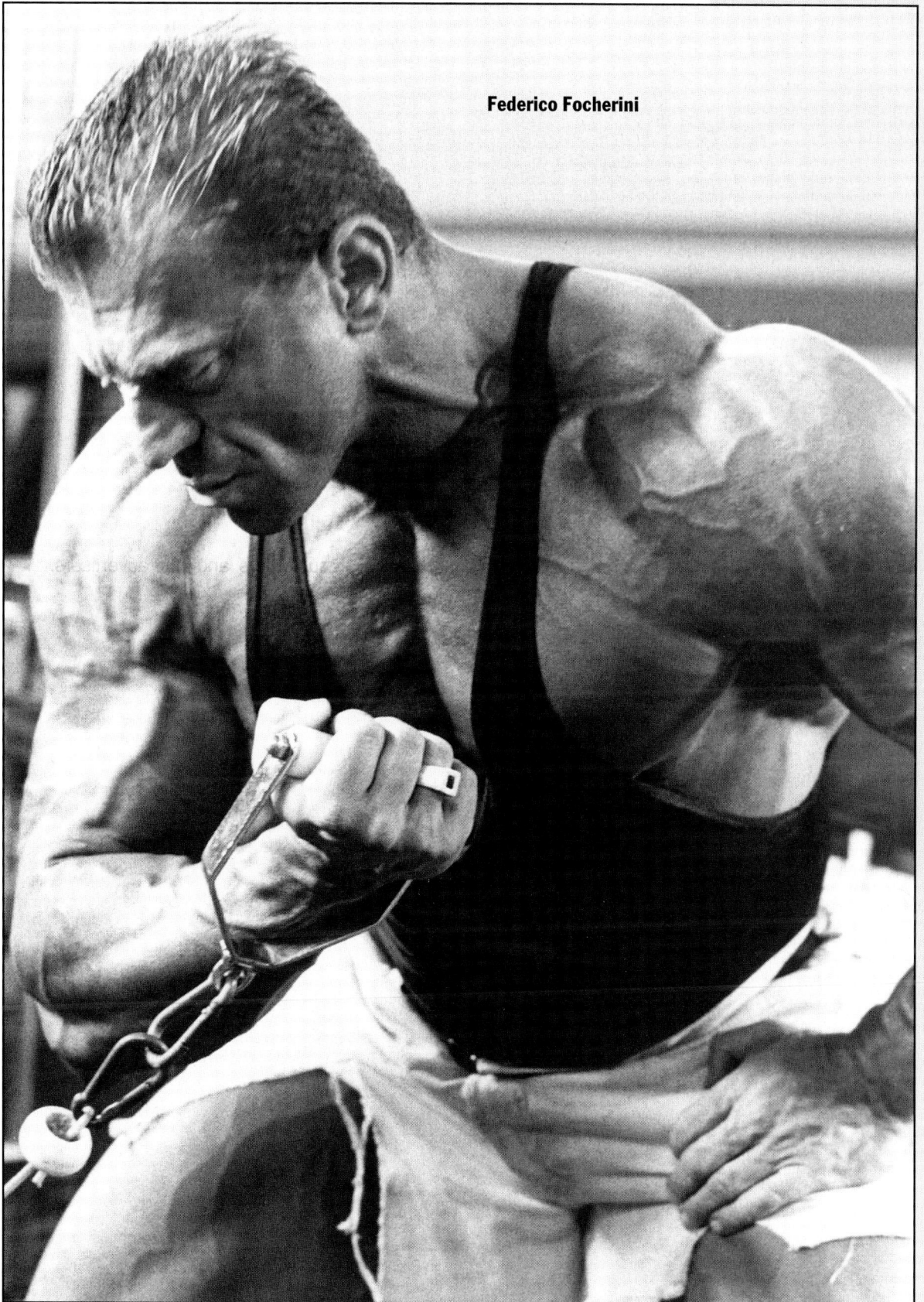

Federico Focherini

THE HEART OF THE SIXTH

During WWII, a battle took place in which over one million men fought and died, and which ultimately decided the course of the war – Stalingrad. Thanks to the incompetence of the Nazi fanatics who had plunged the world into conflict, the entire German Sixth Army was surrounded in the Russian City of Stalingrad (now named Volgograd). The German High Command became alarmed by reports of fit young soldiers who were suddenly dying for no apparent reason. Doctors in the besieged city thawed out frozen bodies in a bunker, and the Luftwaffe flew in pathologists who performed autopsies. It was found that the bone marrow, normally a healthy red or yellow, was a glassy, quivering jelly. The soldiers' hearts were small and brown, with the right ventricle and atrium greatly enlarged. While this is commonly seen in the elderly, in younger populations it is caused by starvation and stress. Daily rations of four ounces of bread and a little horsemeat, plus the stress of months of continuous combat, had in effect aged these soldiers. The condition became known as "The Heart of the

> **"Cheer up Sir, after every December there's always a May."**
>
> – German Soldier at Stalingrad, speaking to his commanding officer. The same soldier then left to take his position, and promptly died for no apparent cause.[1]

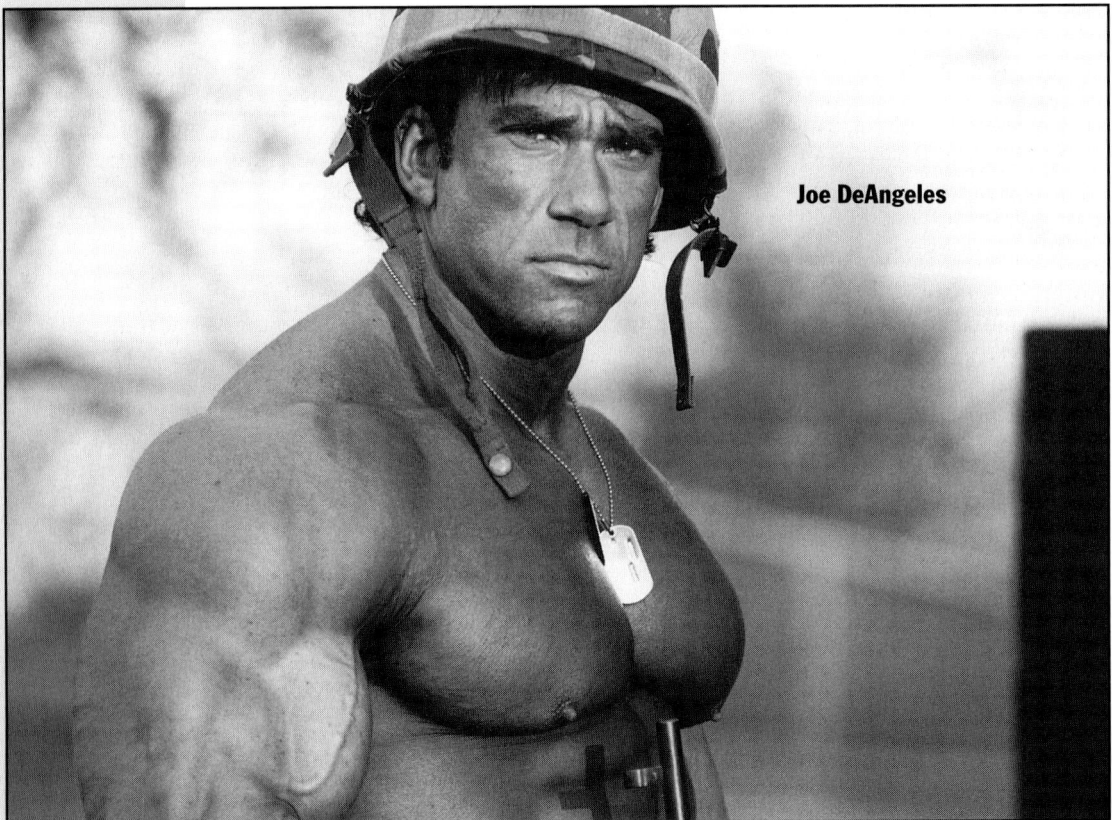

Joe DeAngeles

Sixth Army."[1] Of the 600,000 men who made up the besieged army, 91,000 surrendered, and only 6,000 of the prisoners survived the war. Still, they were more fortunate than most Russian prisoners, of whom only one in 100 returned home.

Why this war story in a bodybuilding book? Because we fear that the Heart of the Sixth is becoming a real threat in hardcore bodybuilding. The continued quest for greater muscle mass and lower fat levels places greater stress on the body (physically, through diet and exercise, and pharmacologically, through the use of drugs such as diuretics and insulin). It has almost certainly led to the deaths of a number of professional body-builders. We lack proof, but those readers who are familiar with our earlier books, will recognize that we are cautious about needlessly ringing alarm bells. We don't write tripe like "Death in the Locker Room." But the reader must remember that overall health is the result of a very delicate metabolic balance. A certain level of bodyfat is healthy, and indeed essential for life itself. The information in this book is powerful, and in the wrong hands, deadly. This is not another legal regurgitation of "for information purposes only." Only a licensed physician may prescribe medication. Only medication obtained from a pharmacist should be used, and preferably while being monitored by health care professionals. And even though you may disagree with a law, that does not justify breaking it. You will find no absolution for such activity in this book. We believe that an informed bodybuilder is a powerful bodybuilder. The only way to change laws and public opinion is through the dissemination of the truth, and engaging others in meaningful dialogue supported by facts, not hype.

We have combed the libraries, scientific journals, bodybuilding magazines and the Internet for the latest information and things that we missed in our previous volume. This book can be considered a comple-mentary book to the first. In other words, if you bought the first don't throw it away, it's still current! This book is going to be controversial, we knew that before it was published. But with more magazines pushing (unrealistically we believe) an all natural format, a large number of bodybuilders were being left out in the cold. That is unfair. Dictating what people may or may not read about in a free society is regressive, and more typical of the deceased Nazi and Soviet regimes. Only 10 years ago, a medical doctor would have been ostracized by his or her colleagues for prescribing alternative health care treatments. Today, doctors routinely refer patients to chiropractors and massage therapists, and prescribe herbal remedies like St. John's Wort. They changed, because the public became more educated about their options, and demanded change. This book is one small step in bringing about further change. Be patient. Use caution. See your physician regularly. And please, take care of yourself, no one in a well-nourished society needs to die from the Heart of the Sixth.

Gerard Thorne and Phil Embleton

Reference
Hymel, K. *Heart of the Sixth Army*, http:www.thehistorynet.com/WorldWarII/articles/1997/11972_side.htm.

CHAPTER ONE

Anabolic Steroids

Despite the new drugs and supplements that have come on the scene over the last 10 years, anabolic steroids still remain the most popular ergogenic aid. Even the new supplements use the words anabolic and steroid-like frequently in their advertising. The manufacturers know that such terms grab bodybuilders' attention like no other. Anti-steroid groups still preach about their evils, but the fact remains that despite over 50 years of athletic use, the vast majority of steroid users don't develop serious side effects. This is not our opinion, it's medical fact. The authors' have spent over 10 years reading just about every book and article pertaining to steroids. We have yet to see one long-term, large sample, controlled study that shows steroid users have a higher incidence of any serious medical problem versus non-users. Yes, there are case studies, and occasionally some seemingly healthy athlete dies of liver cancer or heart disease, but millions of non-users die of the same ailments. If, and it's a big IF, steroids caused liver cancer and heart disease, then the funeral homes and graveyards should be filled with geriatric athletes. We assure you this is not happening.

So as not to be accused of being pro-steroid, let us say that teenagers should not use anabolic steroids (or for that matter any of the other prescription/illegal drugs discussed in this book). There is medical evidence to suggest steroids can produce physiological and psychological effects in such age groups.

Finally steroids are illegal drugs in many countries. In the United States, possession will get you serious jail-time. In our opinion, someone at the local gym using steroids to change his or her physique, should not be placed in the same legal category as a big-time cocaine dealer. But this is where US laws are headed (in fact have gone in some states). So while the health risks can be avoided by using common sense, the same cannot be said for the long-arm of the law. Please obey the laws in your country.

DRUGS AND CYCLES

Rather than just repeat what was said in the *Anabolic Primer*, we will briefly touch on individual steroids and associated stacking drugs, including information and drugs not included in the first book. Where dns (dosage not specified) is encountered in a drug cycle, an average dose may be substituted.

> "If you find someone who is well connected, there should be little chance of fake steroids. If you buy from a middleman – maybe someone five or 10 levels from the source – then your chances of buying fake steroids may be as high as 90 percent."
>
> – Greg Zulak, regular *MuscleMag* columnist, outlining the odds of buying fake steroids on the black market.

Trade Names: Andriol, Androxen, Undestor, Restandol
Generic Name: Testosterone Undecanoate
Gym Dosage: 160 to 400 mg/day, in 4 divided doses

Comments: A very weak steroid believed to work better if stacked with Deca-durabolin.[6] This drug only stays active in the body for a few hours, which is why it must be taken so often.[7]

Trade Names: Anadrol, Anadrol 50, Hemogenin, Anapolon 50, Oxitosona 50, Androyd, Anasteron, Dynasten, Plenastril, Synasteron, Zenalosyn[39]
Generic Name: Oxymetholone
Gym Dosage: 50 to 100 mg/day

Comments: Highly androgenic, this drug should be used no longer than four weeks, and with Nolvadex or Proviron to cut down on side effects. Most gains are lost after the drug is stopped.[6, 10]

Trade Name: Dynabol 50
Generic Name: Nandrolone Cypionate
Gym Dosage: 50 mg/week, i.m.[37] (intramuscular injection)

Trade Name: Nandrobolin[33]
Generic Name: A blend of 2 steroids:
Nandrolone Cypionate 30 mg/ml and
Methandriol 45 mg/ml
Gym Dosage: 1 to 2 ml/week, i.m.

"Steroids can cause premature closure of the growth plates, and side effects in a teen could be a lot more serious than in an adult."

– Dr. Larry D. Bowers, professor and director of the Athletic Testing and Toxicology Laboratory at Indiana University, Indianapolis, echoing the author's views that teenagers should under no circumstances use anabolic steroids.[18]

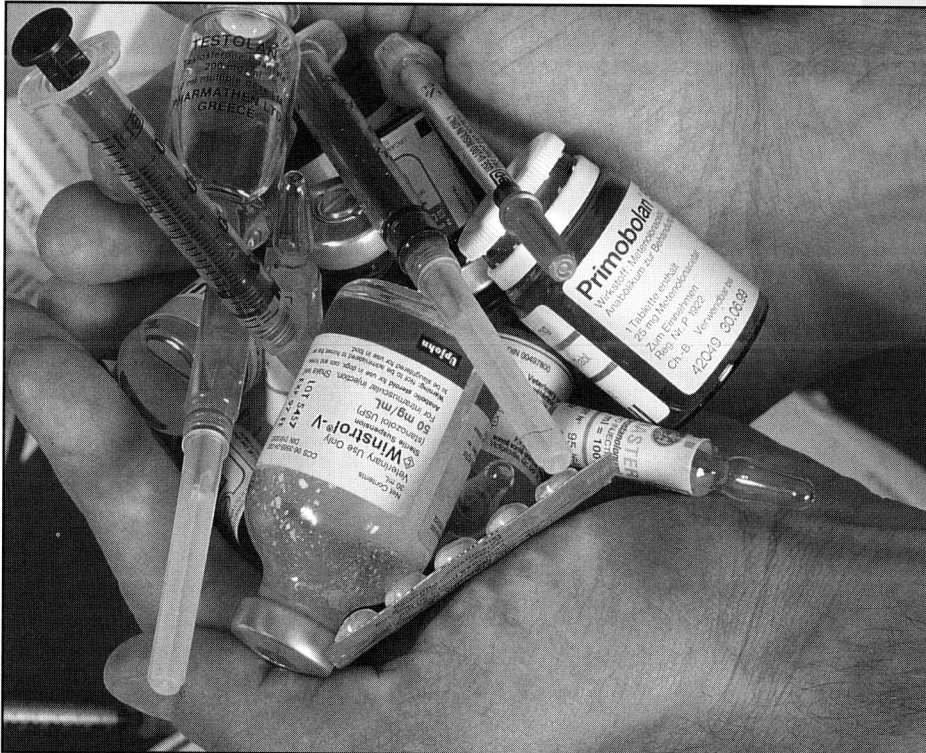

Jean Pierre Fux

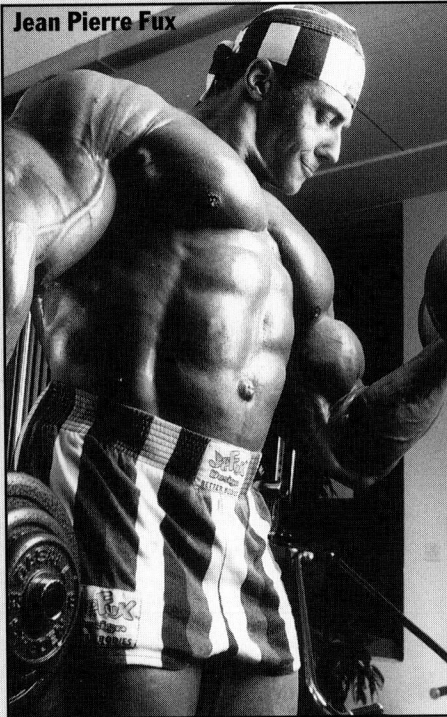

Trade Name: Durabolin
Generic Name: Nandrolone Phenpropionate
Gym Dosage: 100 to 200 mg twice weekly, i.m.

Comments: Faster acting than Deca-Durabolin, but does not stay in the body as long. This drug is considered to be both effective and safe. Stays active in the body for five days.[6,13]

Trade Names: Deca-Durabolin, Deca 50
Generic Name: Nandrolone Decanoate
Gym Dosage: 200 to 800 mg every 1 to 2 weeks

Comments: Voted most likely to fail a drug test, it can be detected in the body a year after last use! It is low in androgenic effects making it popular with female body-builders.[6] Takes three days to dissipate from the injection site and stays active in the body for 17 days.[8] Deca will only convert to estrogen at high doses. This drug produces good size and strength gains. Blood clotting time will be decreased, so dehydrated bodybuilders might experience nosebleeds.[14]

Trade Name: Dynabolon
Generic Name: Nandrolone Undecanoate[34]
Gym Dosage: 2 to 4 cc/week, 80.5 mg/cc

Comments: This drug is similar to Deca-Durabolin, but it is slightly more androgenic. It produces dramatic increases in size and strength.[14]

Trade Name: Finajet
Generic Name: Trenbolone
Gym Dosage: 1 injection every 3 days

Comments: Fast acting drug that gives muscles a hard and cut look. Injection sites can become painful.[14]

Trade Names: Halotestin, Ora-Testryl, Android-F[39]
Generic Name: Fluoxymesterone
(a derivative of methyltestosterone)
Gym Dosage: 10 to 20 mg/day, orally

HA!

Comments: Highly androgenic, this drug should be avoided by females. Known for causing aggressiveness, it should not be taken for longer than four weeks. This drug is used to make already lean muscles look harder and to increase strength.[14] While it is of more benefit to powerlifters and football players, it is a very toxic drug that can make a person go nuts.[27] Because of the risk of increased aggression levels, it is not advisable to use this drug with other steroids.

Trade Names: Laurabolin 50, Fortabol
Generic Name: Nandrolone Laureate
Gym Dosage: 200 to 800 mg every 2 weeks or
100 to 300 mg every 3 days

Comments: It stays active in the body for a month, longer than Deca-durabolin, but Laurabolin is also slower acting.[6, 26]

Trade Names: Cyclomen, Danocrine
Generic Name: Danazol
Gym Dosage: 200 to 800 mg/day, divided into 4
equal doses, orally

Comments: High in androgenic effects.

Trade Names: Maxibolin, Nitrotain [33]
Generic Name: Ethylestrenol
Gym Dosage: 20 to 40 mg/day, orally

Comments: Very popular with female bodybuilders because this drug is low in androgenic effects. Good muscle gains when combined with other steroids. Minimal side effects, but at high dosages it can be toxic to the liver.[36]

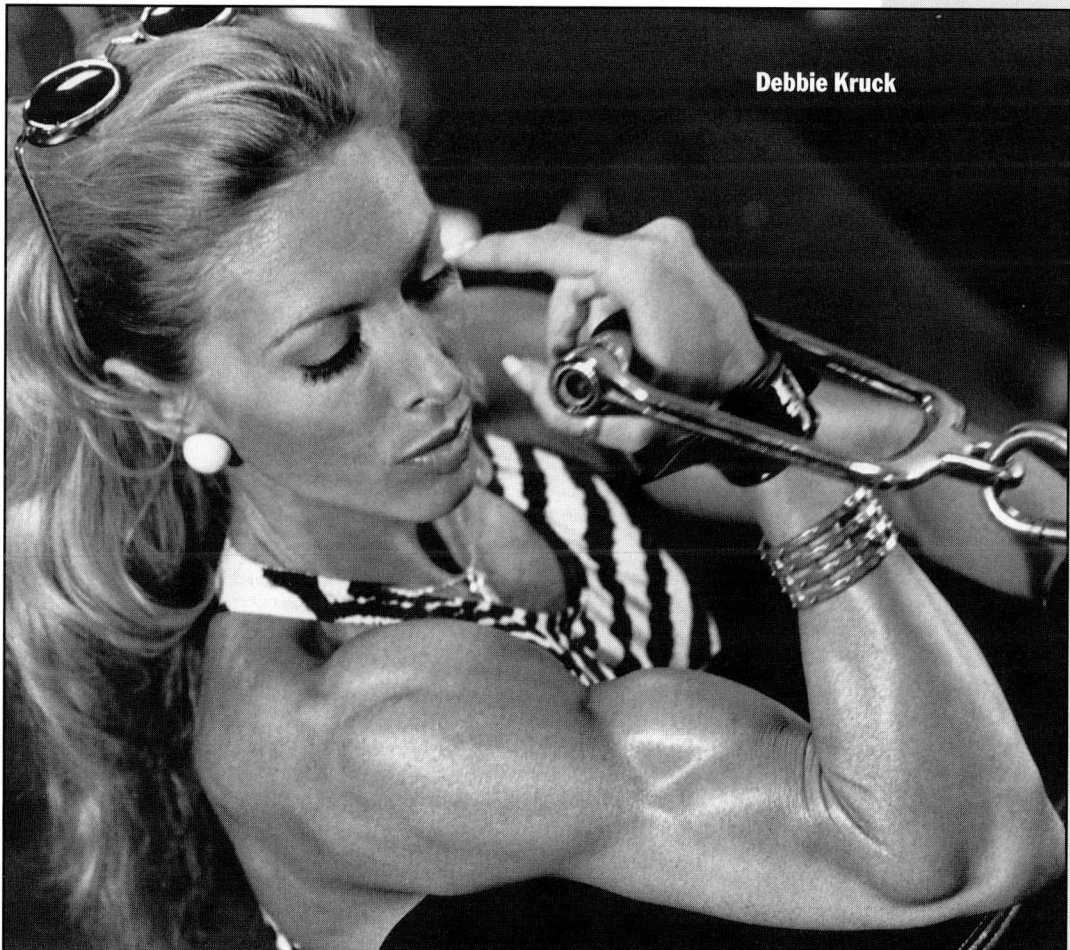

Debbie Kruck

John Brown

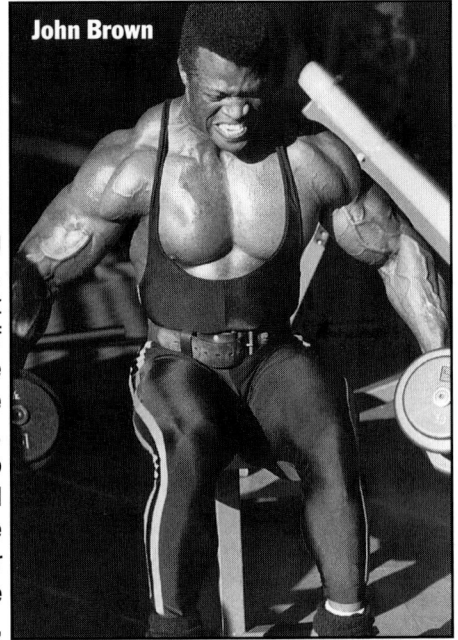

Trade Name: Escilene
Generic Name: Formebolone
Gym Dosage: 1 to 2 ml per bodypart,
injected as needed

Comments: This drug is used to help sagging parts before a competition (or as rumor has it, ensuring that the glove won't fit in prominent criminal cases). It causes swelling at the site of injection, which lasts from 20 to 30 hours. The drug has a painkiller in it to ease soreness. The muscle gains additional definition and hardness. This drug is reported to be only effective in two muscle groups at a time. Escilene is also used as a plateau-buster. Using cell memory, once the swelling goes down, over time and with proper training, the muscle can attain the size it once had. Other than some temporary soreness, there are no side effects.[14, 15]

Trade Names: Equipoise, Ganabol, Boldebol-H, Boldenone 50 [33]
Generic Name: Boldenone Undecylenate
Gym Dosage: 150 to 300 mg/week, i.m. every other day

Comments: Very good mass and strength drug. It has strong androgenic properties and should be combined with Nolvadex.[14, 16]

Trade Name: Drive [33]
Generic Name: A blend of 2 steroids:
         Boldenone 25 mg/ml and
         Methandriol 50 mg/ml
Gym Dosage: 2 ml/week, i.m.[37]

Trade Names: Masteron, Masteril, Drolban, Masterid,
         Mastisol, Metormon, Permastril, Dromostanolone [39]
Generic Name: Drostanolone Propionate
Gym Dosage: 100 mg every 3 days, i.m.

Comments: Being a synthetic derivative of dihydrotestosterone, it will not aromatize at any dosage! Strong anabolic, has anti-estrogenic properties, few reported side effects, and makes muscles look defined and hard. Clears the system 12 days after injection.[25]

Trade Name: Primobolan Depot
Generic Name: Methenolone Acetate
Gym Dosage: 100 to 300 mg/week, orally; 200 to 300 mg/week i.m.

Comments: Popular with females because of its low androgenic effects.[6] It is reported by bodybuilders that much of the gains obtained from this drug are permanent. Primobolan will not aromatize and is not toxic.[23]

Trade Names: Filybol, Orabol-H, Methandriol, Methasus 50[33]
Generic Name: Methandriol
Gym Dosage: 150 mg/day

Comments: Methandriol is the oral, 17-alpha alkylated version of 5-androstenediol.[35] It is highly anabolic and androgenic. It will aromatise and it is moderately toxic. This drug is used for mass and strength gains. One theory holds that Methandriol enhances receptor stimulation, causing the steroid it is stacked with to bind better to androgen sites on the cell.[36]

Trade Name: Spectriol
Generic Name: A blend of 6 steroids:
    Methandriol 20 mg/ml,
    Nandrolone Phenylpropionate 15mg/ml,
    Testosterone Hexahydrobenzoate 10mg/ml,
    Testosterone Enanthate 10mg/ml,
    Testosterone Propionate 5mg/ml and
    Testosterone Cypionate 5mg/ml
Gym Dosage: 1 to 4 ml/week, i.m.

Trade Name: Tribolin 75
Generic Name: A blend of 2 steroids:
    Methandriol 40 mg/ml
    Nandrolone Decanoate 35 mg/ml
Gym Dosage: 3 ml/day, i.m.

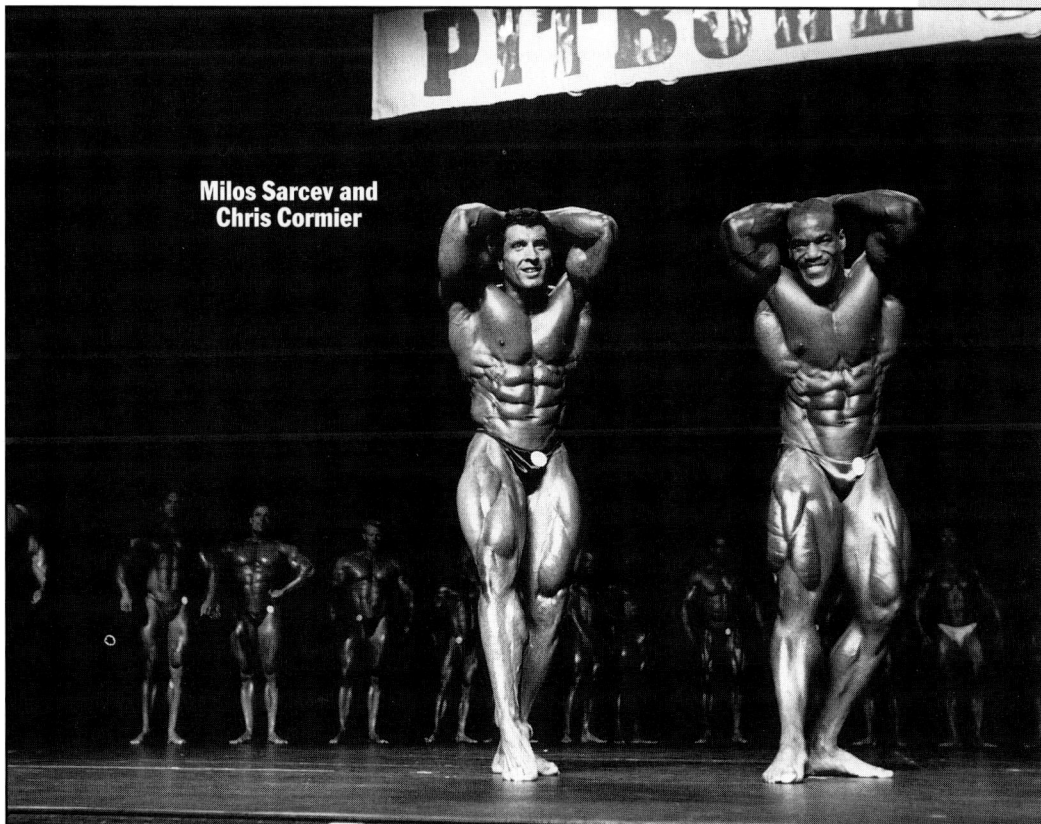

Milos Sarcev and Chris Cormier

> Trade Name: Prodiol (formerly Pentabol)
> Generic Name: A blend of 2 steroids:
> 5-Androstenediol (50 mg) and
> Lysophosphatidylcholine (LPC)(200 mg)
> Gym Dosage: 150 mg/day, orally

Comments: In order to allow for maximum absorption and minimum breakdown of 5-Androstenediol, LPC is used as an absorption agent. Side effects are minimal, because 5-Androstenediol can act as a weak estrogen and bind to the estrogen receptor, preventing stronger estrogens from exerting an effect. It is not recognized by the United States DEA as being an anabolic steroid, because it is naturally occurring. Therefore this is the only steroid on our list that is legal.[35] (See also Testosterone Precursors.)

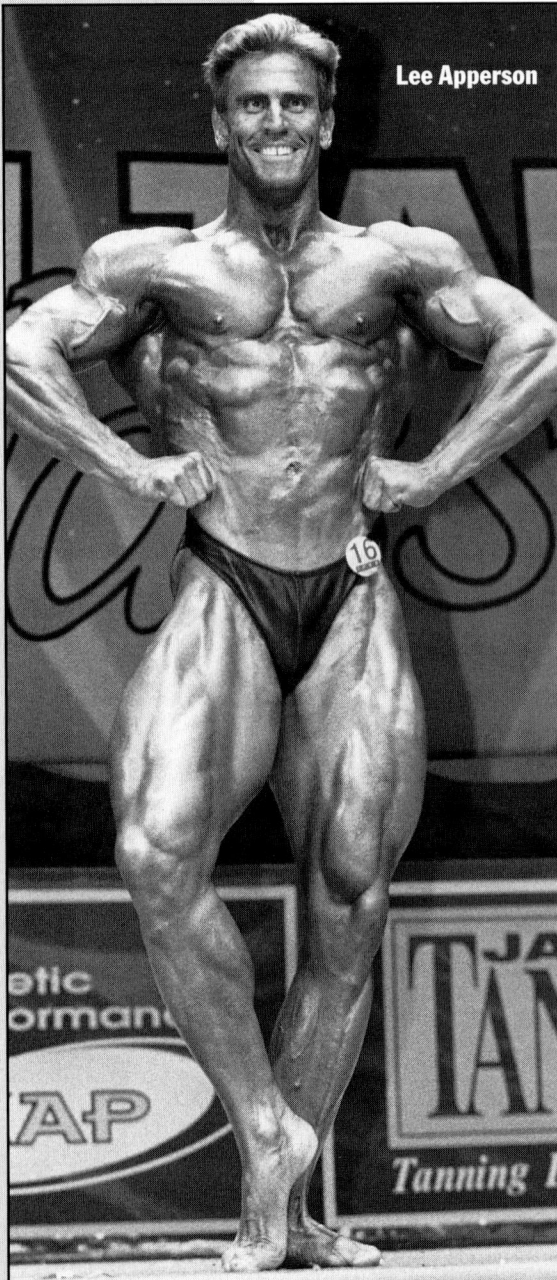

Lee Apperson

> Trade Names: Dianabol, D-bol,
> Danabol, Metabolina,
> Nerobol, Reforvit,
> Pronabol 5,[34] Metaboline[39]
> Generic Name: Methandrostenalone
> Gym Dosage: 15 to 35 mg/day; or
> 20 to 30 mg/day; or 100 mg/day,
> orally; or 50 to 100 mg/week i.m.

Comments: Probably the most popular steroid ever invented. It was developed in the mid-40s and experimentally used on returning POWS who had been on starvation diets.[14] Almost everyone experiences results with this drug. Dramatic strength and size gains are the norm. Gossip has it that a famous bodybuilder with a German accent built his muscles using a combination of Dianabol and Primobolan Depot. Due to problems in obtaining needles, Reforvit has an advantage over other injectables, you can drink it with out much loss of effectiveness. This brand has 25 mg/ml, meaning that a 50 ml bottle is the equivalent of 250 tablets.[6,12] It is highly androgenic, and may cause insomnia at high dosages.[14]

> Trade Name: Cheque Drops
> Generic Name: Mibolerone
> Gym Dosage: A few drops, sub-lingual,
> for a maximum of 2 weeks
> (In dogs, 30 micrograms per 11 kg[5])

Comments: Veterinary steroid used to prevent female dogs from going into heat. Mibolerone blocks the release of LH by the pituitary and prevents complete development of the follicle. Thus ovulation does not occur.[4] In rats, mibolerone is 41 times as an anabolic and 16 times as androgenic as methyltestosterone.[5] This is the most toxic androgenic steroid used. Both boxers and powerlifters use it to increase strength and aggression. It gets into the system within minutes, and has been known to cause users to go nuts (there is even speculation it may cause ear-nibbling among boxers). Lots of side effects, but very slight gains. Most body-builders have nothing to gain by using it. Because of the aggression factor, it should not be used with any other steroids.[28]

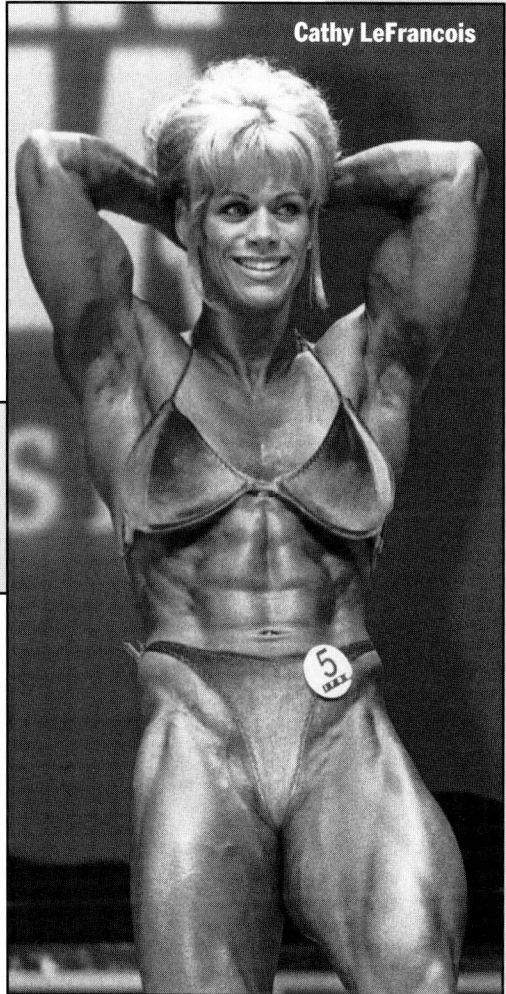

Cathy LeFrancois

Trade Names: Android, Methandren, Testred, Methyltestosterone Tabs, Geri-Bons, Geri-tabs, Dermonal[39]
Generic Name: Methyltestosterone
Gym Dosage: 20 to 50 mg/day, orally

Comments: This drug takes about 30 minutes to get into the system, and is probably second only to Cheque Drops in promoting aggression. The effect lasts for about an hour and a half, leading to workouts that are very intense. This moti-vating factor is about all that can be said about this drug. It is highly androgenic, aromatizes easily and belongs to the 17-alpha-group of steroids which will cause mildly elevated liver function tests. Because of the aggression factor, it should not be used as part of any steroid stack.[14, 36]

Trade Names: Oxandrin, Anavar, Antitriol, Lonovar
Generic Name: Oxandrolone
Dosage: 10 to 20 mg/day for women, 20 to 80 mg/day for men
or 7.5 to 15 mg/day regardless of sex

Comments: Popular with female bodybuilders because it is non-androgenic. Produces a lean and hard look and is ideal for contest preparation. As this drug does not suppress testosterone production, it is often used at the end of a cycle, eliminating the need for HCG or Clomid afterwards.[6, 9]

Trade Name: Parabolan, Finaject[39]
Generic Name: Trenbolone Hexahydrobenzylcarbonate
Gym Dosage: 76 to 152 mg/week; or 152 to 304 mg/week, i.m.

Comments: Powerful drug that builds mass and strength. Very high in androgenic effects.[6] It is a favorite of pre-contest bodybuilders because of its ability to produce dramatic hardness in muscles that are already lean. Parabolan does not aromatize, but it is fairly toxic.[24]

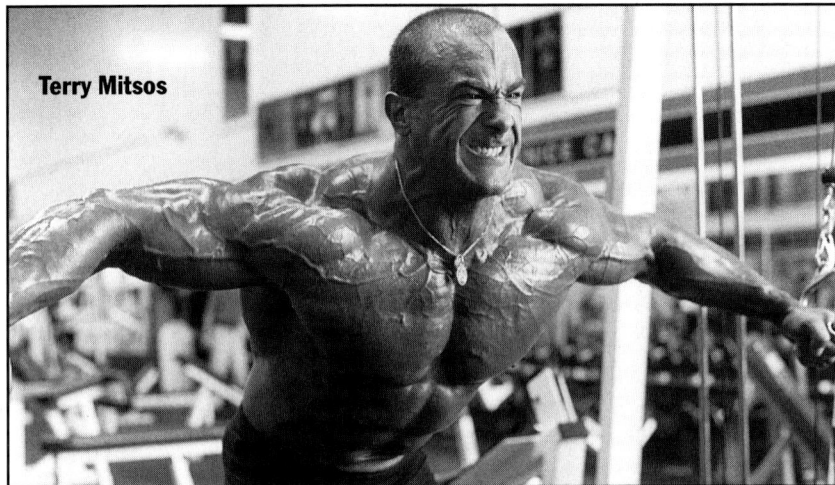

Terry Mitsos

Trade Names: Sustanon 250, Sostenon 250
Generic Name: A blend of 4 steroids:
    Testosterone Propionate (30 mg),
    Testosterone Phenylpropionate (60 mg),
    Testosterone Isocaporate (60 mg) and
    Testosterone Decanoate (100 mg)
Dosage: 1 to 4 cc/week

Comments: This is a very popular drug, because it is easily obtainable and really a pre-packaged drug cycle. Each component has a specific length of time in which it remains active in the body: Propionate, three to four days; Phenylpropionate and Isocaporate, one to three weeks; and Decanoate, two to four weeks. Because of the retention time, it is not necessary to take large doses. This blend is a mass building drug, which is also self-tapering. It is recommended for a ski-slope cycle.[6, 14]

Trade Name: Omnadren
Generic Name: A blend of 4 steroids:
    Testosterone Propionate,
    Testosterone Phenpropionate,
    Testosterone Isohexanate and
    Testosterone Hexanoate
Gym Dosage: 1 to 4 cc/week

Comments: A mass and strength building drug. More androgenic than Sustanon.[6]

Trade Names: Winstrol, Winstrol-V, Stanabol, Stanazol, Stanosus,[33] Stromba, Strombaject[39]
Generic Name: Stanazolol
Gym Dosage: 50 mg/day, i.m.; or 6 mg/day, orally

Comments: Produces mild gains and has few side effects. It is known for increasing stamina. It must be injected daily, which for most people is an inconvenience.[14, 38] Stanazol is the drug made famous by Canadian sprinter Ben Johnson's positive drug test at the 1988 Seoul Olympics.

Trade Name: Sten
Generic Name: A blend of 100 mg Testosterone and 20 mg DHEA
Gym Dosage: 360 to 480 mg/week, i.m.

Comments: A good drug to add to a bulking cycle. It is in fact a weaker version of Sostenon 250, but with worse side effects because of the high amount of DHT present.[14, 20]

Trade Names: Testosus 100, Testosterone Suspension,[33]
Malogen, Delatestryl, Neo-pause,
PMS-testosterone Enanthate, Duogex,
Climacteron, Orchisterone-P, Anadiol, Anatest[39]
Generic Name: Testosterone Suspension
Gym Dosage: 100 mg every other day, i.m.

Comments: Stays active in the body for one day. Highly androgenic, but a good mass and strength building drug.[6]

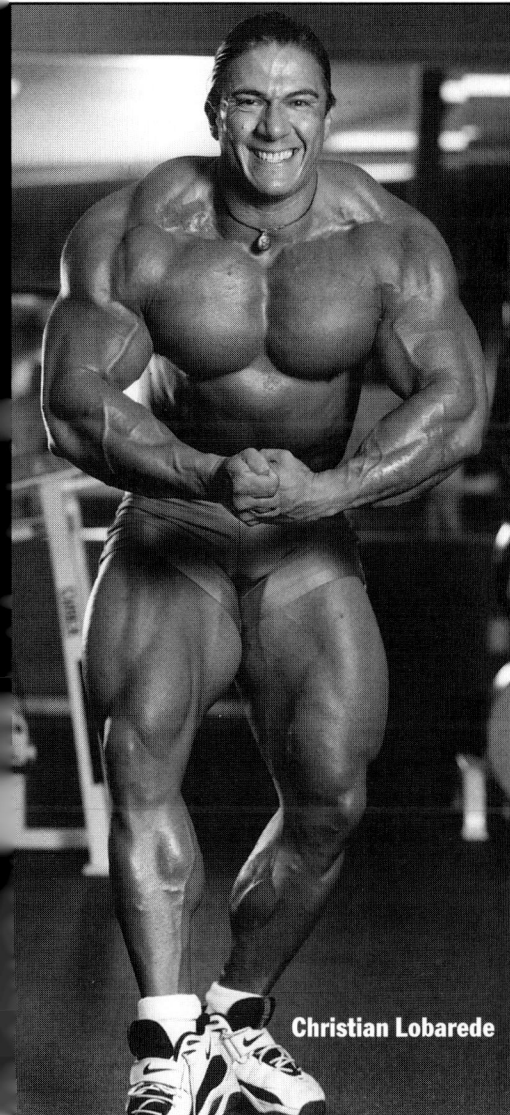

Christian Lobarede

Trade Names: Testoviron,
Testex, Supertest,
Tepro Sterile Injection,[33]
Virormone[34]
Generic Name: Testosterone Propionate
Gym Dosage: 100 to 200 mg every 3 days; or 250 to 500 mg/week, i.m.

Comments: Stays active in the body for three to five days. Same comments as Suspension.[6] Injection site tends to be painful.[18]

Trade Names: Depo-Testosterone,
Testo La, Cooper's Banrot[33]
Generic Name: Testosterone Cypionate
Gym Dosage: 200 to 600 mg/week

Comments: Stays active in the body from one to three weeks. Same comments as Suspension.[6, 19]

Trade Names: Testoviron Depot,
Testosterona 200,
Ringer Testosterone,[33]
Androtardyl,
Testex Leo Prolongatum[34]
Generic Name: Testosterone Enanthate
Gym Dosage: 200 to 600 mg every 10 to 14 days, i.m.

Comments: Stays active in the body from two to four weeks. Same comments as Suspension.[6] Those who don't like needles will like this drug, because of the infrequency of the shots.[17]

Trade Name: Primoteston Depot 250
Generic Name: Testosterone Enanthate
Gym Dosage: 250 to 500 mg/week, i.m.

Comments: Same as Suspension.[21]

Trade Names: Finaplex-S, Finaplex-H
Generic Name: Trenbolone Acetate Cattle Implants
Strength: 20mg trenbolone acetate per pellet.
Gym Dosage: 30 to 60 mg every other day, i.m. or absorbed through skin

Comments: Strong anabolic/androgenic. Very good fat-burner. Unlike other implants, it does not contain estradiol. Reported to be very hard on the kidneys. Like all cattle implants, bodybuilders grind the pills and either inject or combine it with dimethyl sulfoxide (DMSO) and water, and then absorb the drug through the skin.[30] This is not something we recommend, but that's what some people do.

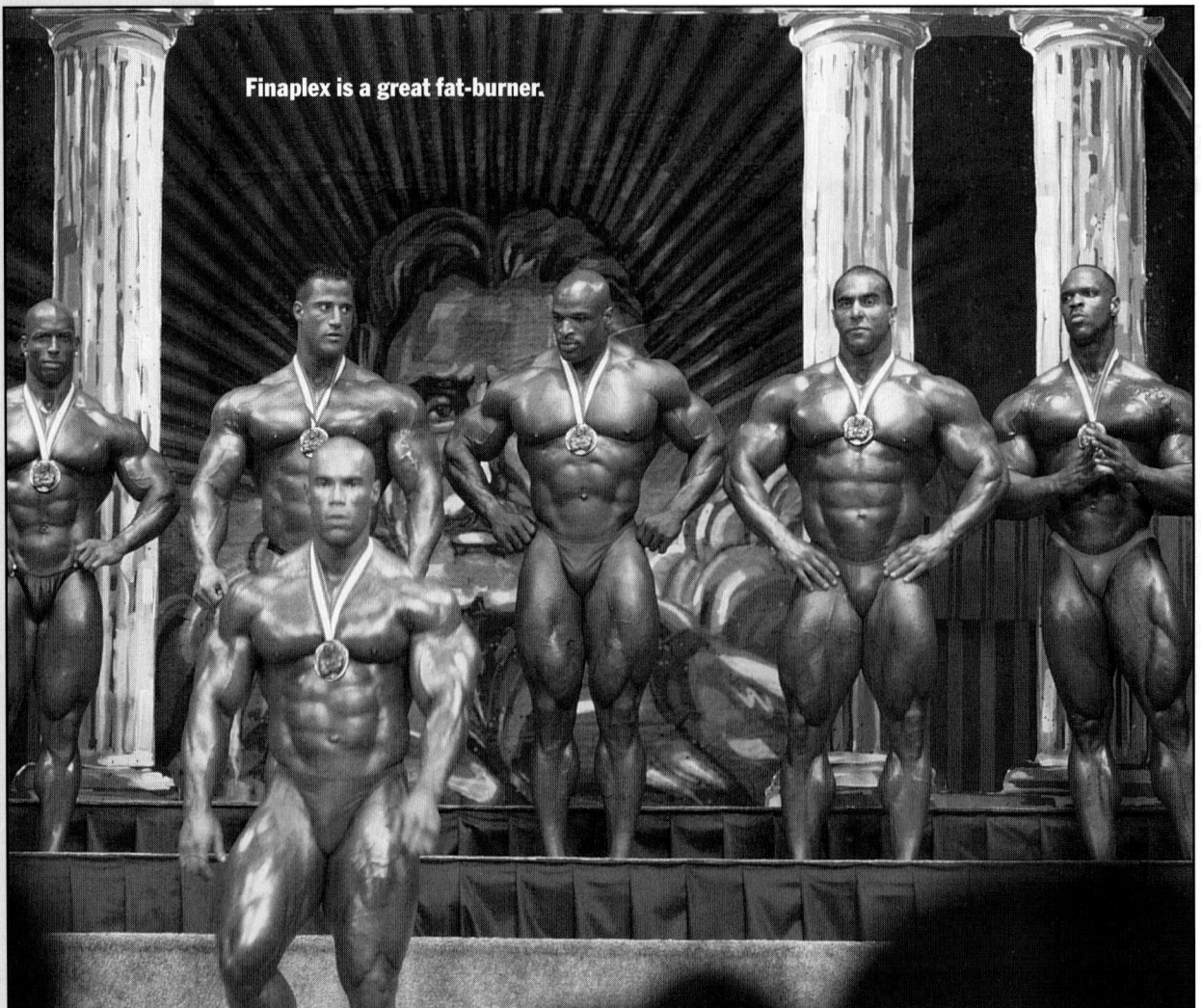

Finaplex is a great fat-burner.

Trade Names: Revalor, Revalor-S
Generic Name: Trenbolone Acetate/ Estradiol Cattle Implants
Strength: 20 mg trenbolone acetate and 20 mg estradiol per pellet
Gym Dosage: 30 to 60 mg every other day, i.m.; or absorbed through the skin

Comments: Has the same properties as other Trenbolone Acetate implants, bodybuilders chemically remove the estradiol. Very good mass-building drug.[31]

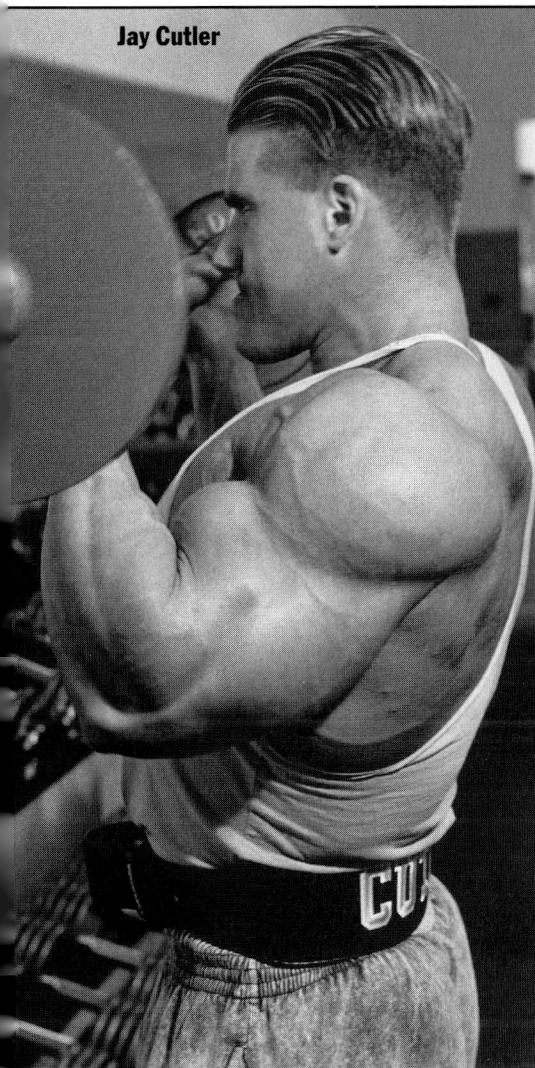

Jay Cutler

Trade Names: Synovex-H, Implus
Generic Name: Testosterone Propionate/Estradiol Benzoate Cattle Implants
Strength: 200 mg testosterone propionate and 20 mg estradiol per pellet
Gym Dosage: 50 to 100 mg every other day, i.m. or absorbed through the skin

Comments: Same filtration process as Revalor.[32]

Trade Name: Ralgrow
Generic Name: Zeranol Cattle Implants
Strength: 72 mg Zeranol per pellet.
Gym Dosage: 30 to 60 mg every other day, i.m.; or absorbed through the skin

Comments: Reportedly doesn't work in humans.[29]

Trade Name: Proviron
Generic Name: Masterolone
Gym Dosage: 25 to 50 mg/ day;
or 50 mg twice/day, orally

Comments: Very weak anabolic steroid that produces a hard, dense look to the muscles. It is primarily used in a stack because of its antiestrogenic properties.[6] Mainly used by bodybuilders to restore libido and sexual function, which may be decreased during a long steroid cycle. It does not increase testosterone production, nor will it help in maintaining strength and mass gains after a cycle.[22]

Trade Names: Ardomon, Clom 50, Clomid, Clomifen, C-ratioph, Clomiphen-Merck, Clomipheni citras, Clomivid, Clostilbegyt, Dufine, Dyneric, Gravosan, Indovar, Klomifen, Kyliformon, Omifin, Pergotime, Pioner, Prolifen, Serofene, Serophene, Serpafar, Tokormon.
Generic Name: Clomiphene Citrate[1]
Gym Dosage: 50 to 100 mg/day, orally, with meals[2]

Comments: Clomiphene is a non-steroidal agent which may induce ovulation in unovulatory women (it's a fertility drug). This response to cyclic clomiphene therapy appears to be mediated through increased output of pituitary gonadotrophins. This in turn stimulates the maturation and endocrine activity of the ovarian follicle, and the subsequent development and function of the corpus luteum. The role of the pituitary is indicated by increased urinary estrogen excretion. Antagonism of competitive inhibition of endogenous estrogen may play a role in the action of clomiphene on the pituitary.[1]

Clomiphene's ability to act as an antiestrogenic cuts down on side effects like gynecomastia. Further, this drug causes an elevation of follicle stimulating hormone (FSH) and luteinizing hormone (LH). This increases natural testosterone production. Once a bodybuilder comes off a cycle, production has already been shut down. Problems of impotence, depression, mass and strength loss may all occur. Some bodybuilders choose to remain on a cycle indefinitely, rather than experience these side effects. Clomiphene reduces the group of side effects, collectively known as the Steroid Crash. Normally, bodybuilders will take the gym dosage for a two-week period after coming off a cycle. NOTE – be aware that there are some serious side effects with this drug. Blurring and other visual problems can occur (particularly in variable lighting), making driving and operating heavy machinery more hazardous than usual. If you are using steroids that are hard on the liver, or you've suffered from liver disease, we advise you to avoid this drug. Female bodybuilders are at risk for multiple pregnancy and ovarian cysts. Other less frequently reported symptoms include: nausea, vomiting, increased nervous tension, depression, fatigue, dizziness, insomnia, headache, breast soreness, heavier menses, intermenstrual spotting, allergic dermatitis, weight gain, increased urinary frequency or volume (a serious issue if combined with diuretics), and moderate, reversible hair loss. The therapeutic dose for this drug is a maximum of 100 mg/day for five days. The safety of long-term cyclic use has not been established.[1]

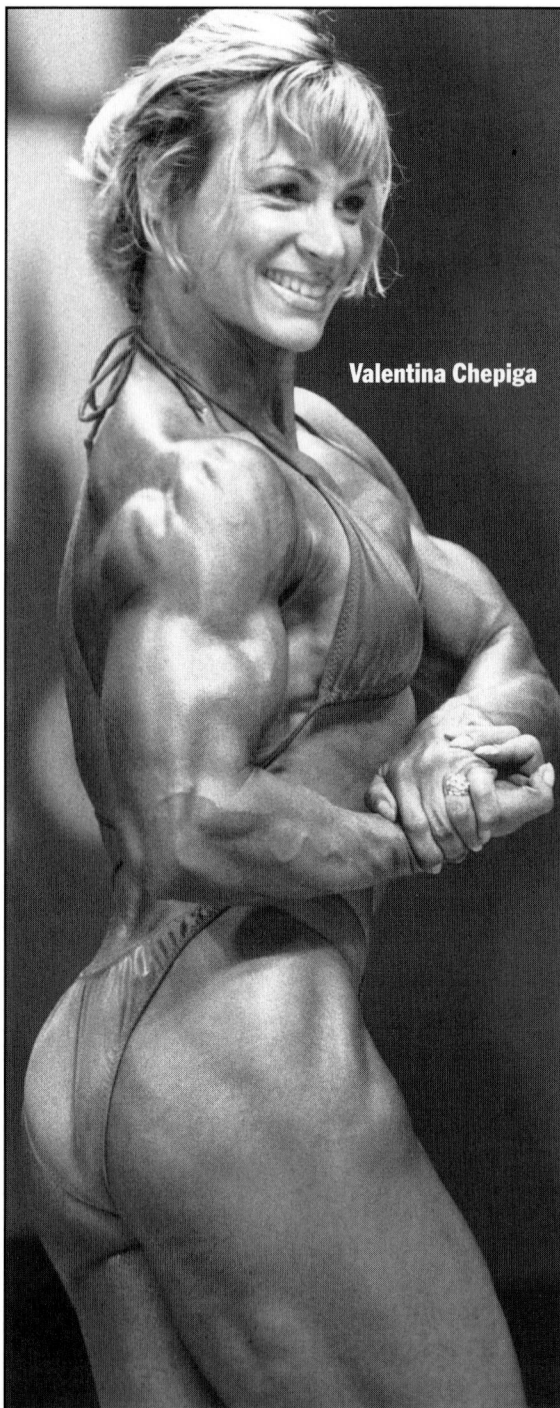

Valentina Chepiga

Trade Names: Sexovid, Rehibin, Ondogyne, Neoclym, Fertodur
Generic Name: Cyclofenil
Gym Dosage: 400 to 600 mg/day

Comments: This is a weak estrogen that works as an anti-estrogen, by binding to estrogen receptors to prevent stronger estrogens from exerting their effects. Cyclofenil is also a testosterone booster, similar in action to HCG, Clomid and Proviron. At a dosage of 100mg, it can double endogenous levels of testosterone. It reduces water retention and makes the muscles appear harder. Cyclofenil is effective at preventing the loss of strength associated with the end of a cycle. Slight gains is size and strength, boosted energy levels and a faster recovery rate are also experienced with this drug.[11]

Trade Name: Nolvadex, Nolvadex-D (1)
Generic Name: Tamoxifen Citrate
Gym Dosage: 10 to 20 mg/day[3]

Comments: Tamoxifen is a nonsteroidal agent that has demonstrated potent antiestrogenic properties. These effects are related to its ability to compete with estrogen for binding sites in target tissues such as the breast. It is effective in significantly lowering the recurrence of breast cancer in estrogen receptor positive tumors.[1] This ability to target breast tissue also makes it the drug of choice for male bodybuilders. It prevents gynecomastia, among other side effects. It is generally taken both during the steroid cycle and after the cycle (with clomiphene).

Possible adverse side effects include: nausea, vomiting, hot flashes, vaginal bleeding, vaginal discharge and skin rash. Those with any pre-existing liver problem should avoid this drug. Visual problems can arise, and the chances of occurrence increase with dosage and length of time taken.[1] It has been linked to testicular cancer in rats.[6]

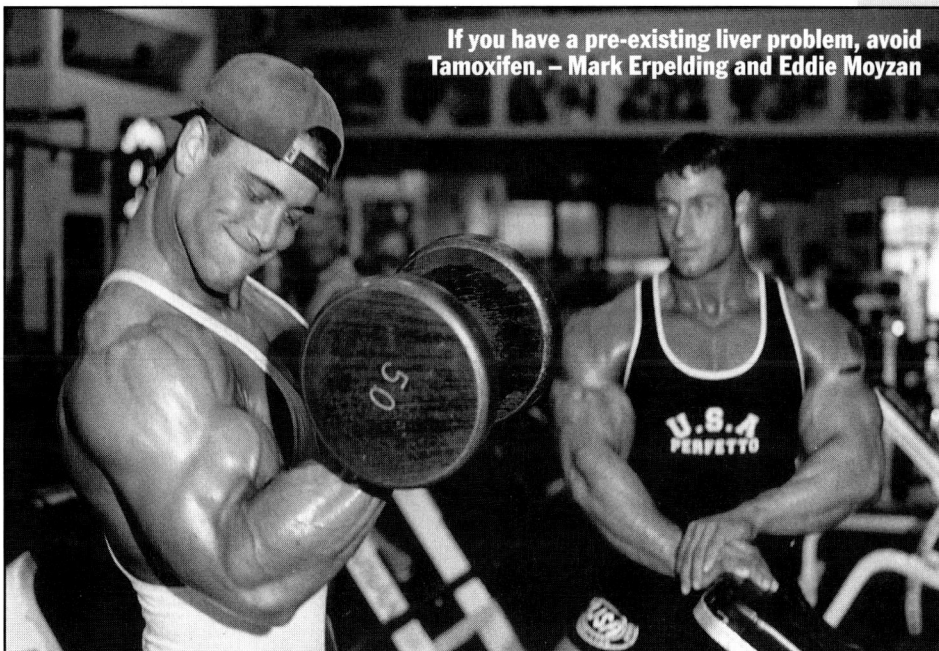

If you have a pre-existing liver problem, avoid Tamoxifen. – Mark Erpelding and Eddie Moyzan

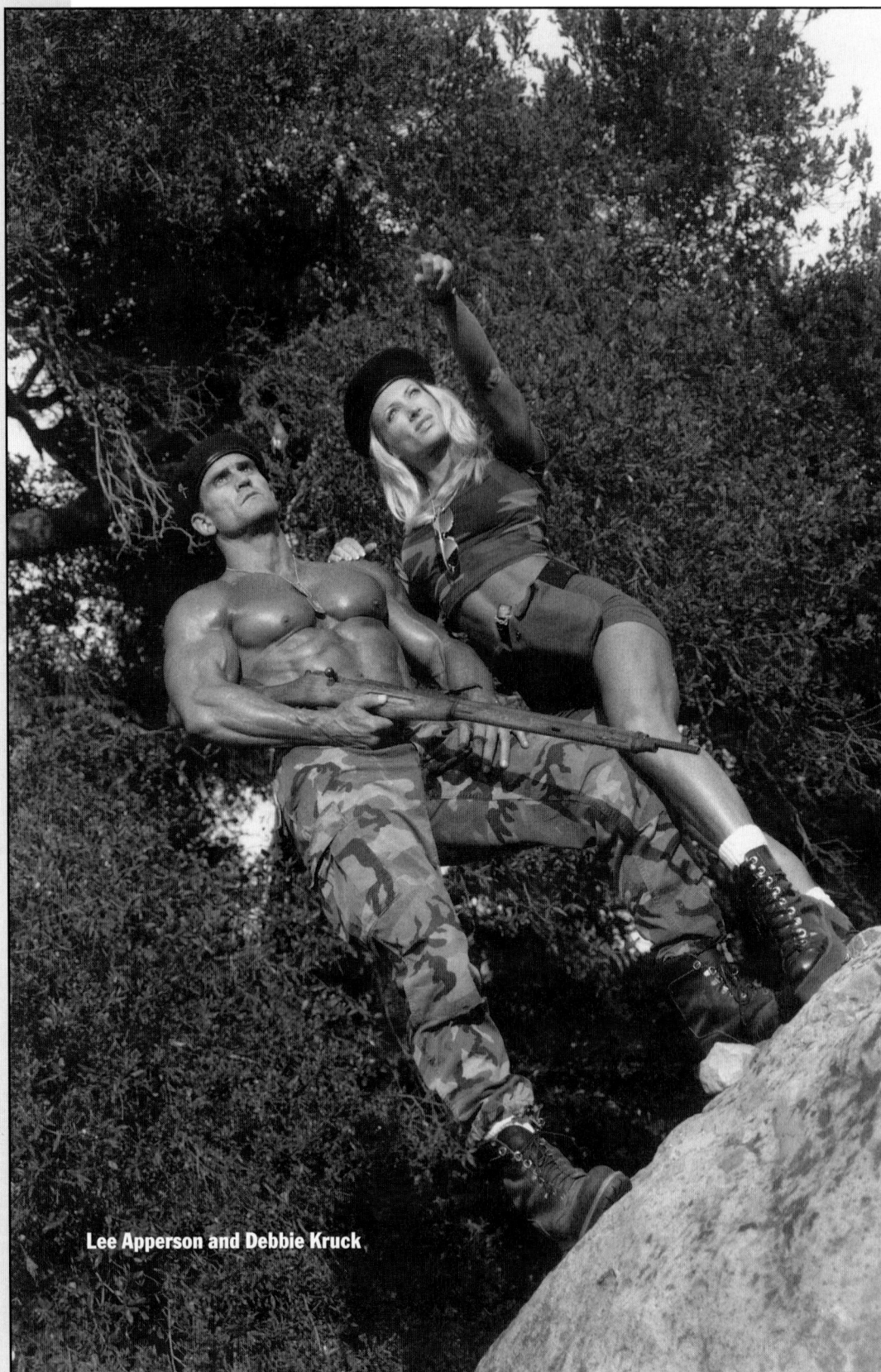

Lee Apperson and Debbie Kruck

References

1) Krogh, C. (Editor-in-Chief). *CPS, Compendium of Pharmaceuticals and Specialties*, Canadian Pharmaceutical Association, Ottawa, Ontario, 1995.
2) Clomid. *Drugs, Absolute Truth Hardcore Bodybuilding*, http://www.geocities.com/HotSprings/2369/newclomid.htm.
3) Nolvadex. *Drugs, Absolute Truth Hardcore Bodybuilding*, http://members.tripod.com~newguru/newnolvadex.html.
4) Wannamaker, B. and Pettes, C. *Applied Pharmacology For The Veterinary Technician*, W.B. Saunders Company, Philadelphia, 1996.
5) Booth, H. and McDonald, L. (eds.). Veterinary Pharmacolgy and Therapeutics, 6th edition, Iowa State University Press, Ames, 1988.
6) David's Steroid Page, http://www.davids-steroidpage.com.
7) Androil, Drugs, *Absolute Truth Hardcore Bodybuilding*, http://members.tripod.com/~newguru/newandroil.html.
8) Deca-Durabolin, Drugs, *Absolute Truth Hardcore Bodybuilding*, http://members.tripod.com~newguru/newdecadurabolin.html.
9) Anavar, Drugs, *Absolute Truth Hardcore Bodybuilding*, http://members.tripod.com/~newguru/newanavar.html.
10) Anadrol, Drugs, *Absolute Truth Hardcore Bodybuilding*, http://members.tripod.com/~newguru/newanadrol.html.
11) Cyclofenil, Drugs, *Absolute Truth Hardcore Bodybuilding*, http://www.geocities.com/HotSprins/2369/newcyclofenil.htm.
12) Dianabol, Drugs, *Absolute Truth Hardcore Bodybuilding*, http://members.tripod.com/~newguru/newdianabol.html
13) Durabolon, Drugs, *Absolute Truth Hardcore Bodybuilding*, http://members.tripod.com/~newguru/newdurabolon.html
14) *Steroid Info*, http://www.student.hro.nl/0519852/roids2.htm.
15) Esiclene, Drugs, *Absolute Truth Hardcore Bodybuilding*, http://members.tripod.com/~newguru/newesiclene.html.
16) Equipoise, Drugs, *Absolute Truth Hardcore Bodybuilding*, http://members.tripod.com/~newguru/newequipoise.html.
17) Test Enanthate, Drugs, *Absolute Truth Hardcore Bodybuilding*, http://members.tripod.com/~newguru/newtestenanthate.html.
18) Test Propinate, Drugs, *Absolute Truth Hardcore Bodybuilding*, http://members.tripod.com/~newguru/newtestpropinate.html.
19) Test Cypionate, Drugs, *Absolute Truth Hardcore Bodybuilding*, http://members.tripod.com/~newguru/newtestcypionate.html.
20) Sten, Drugs, *Absolute Truth Hardcore Bodybuilding*, http://members.tripod.com/~newguru/newsten.html.
21) Primoteston Depot, Drugs, *Absolute Truth Hardcore Bodybuilding*, http://members.tripod.com/~newguru/newprimotestondepot.html.
22) Proviron, Drugs, *Absolute Truth Hardcore Bodybuilding*, http://www.geocities.com/HotSprings/2369/newproviron.htm.
23) Primobolan Depot, Drugs, *Absolute Truth Hardcore Bodybuilding*, http://members.tripod.com/~newguru/newprimobolandepot.html.
24) Parabolan, Drugs, *Absolute Truth Hardcore Bodybuilding*, http://members.tripod.com/~newguru/newparabolan.html.
25) Masteron, Drugs, *Absolute Truth Hardcore Bodybuilding*, http://www.geocities.com/HotSprings/2369/newmasteron.htm.
26) Laurabolin, Drugs, *Absolute Truth Hardcore Bodybuilding*, http://members.tripod.com/~newguru/newlaurabolin.html.
27) Halotestin, Drugs, *Absolute Truth Hardcore Bodybuilding*, http://members.tripod.com/~newguru/newhalotestin.html.
28) Cheque Drops, Drugs, *Absolute Truth Hardcore Bodybuilding*, http://www.geocities.com/HotSprings/2369/newcgequedrops.htm.
29) Ralgrow, Drugs, *Absolute Truth Hardcore Bodybuilding*, http://www.geocities.com/HotSprings/2369/newralgrow.htm.
30) Finaplix, Drugs, *Absolute Truth Hardcore Bodybuilding*, http://www.geocities.com/HotSprings/2369/newfinaplix.htm.
31) Revalor, Drugs, *Absolute Truth Hardcore Bodybuilding*, http://www.geocities.com/HotSprings/2369/newrevalor.htm.
32) Synovex, Drugs, *Absolute Truth Hardcore Bodybuiilding*, http://www.geocities.com/HotSprings/2369/newsynovex.htm.
33) Juice From Down Under, *Absolute Truth Hardcore Bodybuilding*, http://members.tripod.com/~newguru/downundersteroids.htm.
34) European Steroid Cost, *Absolute Truth Hardcore Bodybuilding*, http://members.tripod.com/~newguru/europeansteroidscost.htm.
35) Prodiol, *A Steroid Derivative That Slipped Through*, http://www.massquantities.com/products/prodiol.html.
36) M, http://cpt.pix.za/roids/M.htm.
37) *If I'd Been Smart I Would Have Stopped There, But Being Naturally Greedy (I Remember A Doctor Saying To Me Later That "Nobody Does Just One Course!") I Had To Jab Again*, http://www.anabolicsteroids.com/jabber.html.
38) Winstrol, Drugs, *Absolute Truth Hardcore Bodybuilding*, http://members.tripod.com/~newguru/newwinstrol.html.
39) *IOC Catagories of banned substances*, C. Anabolic Agents E.G., http://www.cces.ca/english/drugfr/b-r-1a3.html.

CHAPTER TWO

Through the Generations with Creatine

In the long history of athletic supplementation few substances have had the impact of creatine. First introduced in 1993, creatine has virtually revolution-ized the supplement industry. Sure, every few years a new fad supplement comes along, but it was creatine that set the standard for things to come.

Unlike most supplements prior to 1993, creatine has the scientific credibility to go with it. Rather than relying on hype and creative advertising, creatine manufacturers used scientific research to establish credibility, and by all accounts they've succeeded. To test creatine's effects, an experiment is set up where half the subjects use the substance and the other half don't (control group). After a given period of time, the subjects are evaluated on a number of tasks involving strength and power. Many athletic supplements fail. But with creatine the users score significantly higher on tests than the control group.

Creatine is a natural substance synthesized from the amino acids arginine, glycine and methionine. In addition to being manufactured by the body, creatine is found in high concentrations in many foods including red meat. Although there's a trace amount stored extracellularly, the vast majority of creatine is stored inside muscle cells. Approximately 40 percent occurs in free form, with the other 60 percent in phosphoralated form. It's the latter form that plays the big role in energy production.

ATP – ENERGY FOR THE AGES

The body's primary source of energy is a compound called adenosine triphosphate – ATP. The adenosine and phosphate groups are held together by high energy bonds. It is the breaking of these bonds, and the subsequent release of stored energy, that powers most of the body's systems. This reaction is summarized as follows:

$$ATP - (ADP + P (phosphate)) + Energy$$

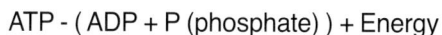

Now here's where creatine comes in. Once taken into muscle cells creatine combines with the free phosphate to form phosphocreatine. Phosphocreatine then serves as a backup source when ATP levels run low. The phosphate part of the compound combines with ADP to form more ATP. The more phosphocreatine available the faster, and ultimately more, ATP generated.

This is just one of creatine's useful effects. It also causes cellular volumization. In short, high creatine levels cause the muscles to absorb and hold more water. Previously flat muscles swell up. And what's nice about the whole process is that the extra water doesn't produce a bloated appearance.

A third benefit to creatine is its effects on strength. Virtually everyone who uses creatine experiences strength increases anywhere from 10 to 30 percent. This effect is probably the least understood of creatine's effects. Some have suggested it's a case of physics not physiology. Larger muscles, due to water retention, may change the body's levers, thus creating superior mechanical advantages. Others suggest increased energy reserves allow the individual to train harder, ultimately producing greater increases in strength. Finally, there may be some unknown intrinsic factor (increased DNA synthesis, strengthened cross-bridges between muscle fibers, etc.) that accounts for the change. Whatever the explanation, athletes welcome the ability to go into the gym and hoist more iron!

CREATINE GENERATIONS

Like most supplements that have staying power, creatine has undergone a sort of supplement evolution, commonly referred to as generations.

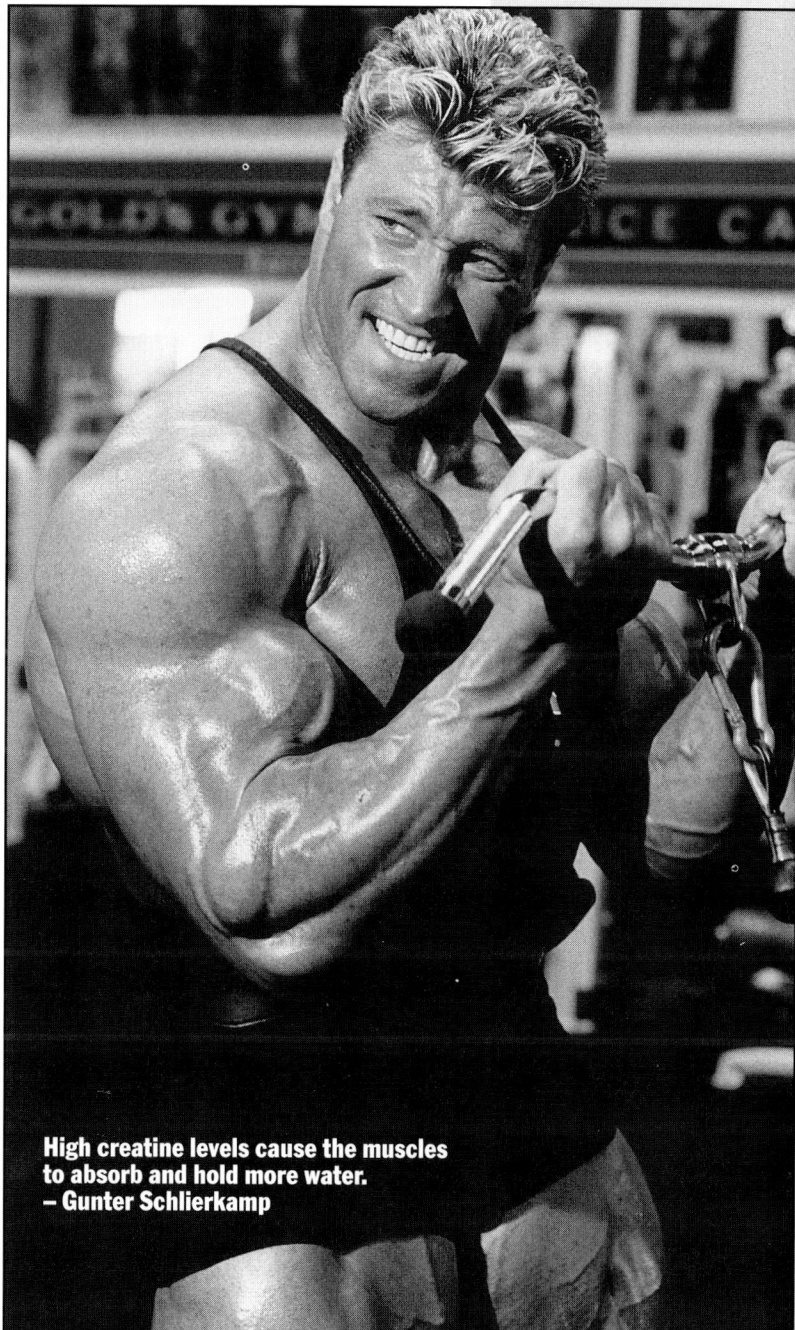

High creatine levels cause the muscles to absorb and hold more water.
– Gunter Schlierkamp

"The reason for Cell-Tech's superior cell volumization effect is primarily due to an ingredient called lipoic acid. It doesn't just cause the pancreas to release insulin, it actually mimics the action of insulin in the body, helping to shuttle more glucose and amino acids into the muscle cells for more muscle growth and better recovery."

– Greg Zulak, *MuscleMag* columnist and MuscleTech spokesman commenting on the first third generation creatine supplement, Muscle Tech's Cell-Tech.

FIRST GENERATION

The vast majority of first generation creatine supplements come as creatine monohydrate – a white crystalline powder. Both characteristics are vital in determining the quality of a given brand. Most cheaper brands are off-white in color and look more like protein powder. Quality brands are pure white. If you see 2000 grams of creatine on sale for $30, we suggest a dose of skepticism. It costs big bucks to produce a quality creatine supplement. There's no way a manufacturer can market a high quality creatine supplement and make a profit at basement bargain prices. We strongly advise spending the extra money and buying quality brands like EAS, TwinLab, MuscleTech or Robert Kennedy's new Formula One Elite Series.

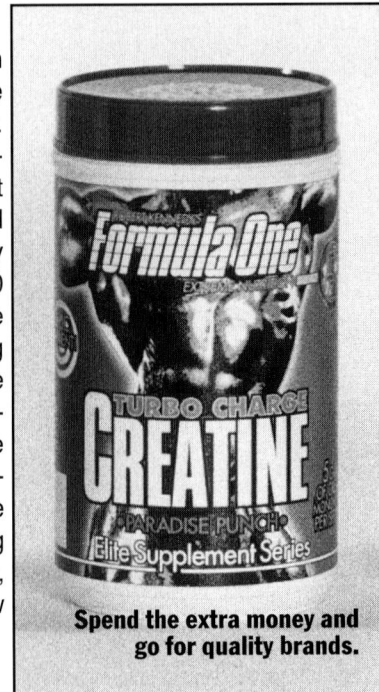

Spend the extra money and go for quality brands.

SECOND GENERATION

Early on, creatine researchers determined that creatine absorption was increased when insulin levels were high. Insulin is the body's primary storage hormone. Besides its role in regulating sugar, it also transports many other substances in and out of the blood stream. Some athletes took the logical step and began using insulin with creatine. We don't advise doing this and we'll say more on insulin later in the chapter. The natural way to do things is to stimulate insulin production by combining creatine with a simple sugar source. EAS was the first major player on the scene with their Phospagen HP creatine, but now the market is flooded with such second generation products.

Before we move on to third generation creatine supplements we should update you on a new research that may improve your creatine usage. A recent study in *Science News* found that when nutrients are mixed with grapefruit juice, absorption goes up by a factor of four. Grapefruit contains a compound called bergmottin that interferes with the enzymes that breakdown many drugs and nutrients before they have a chance to be absorbed.[5] Whether the same would hold true for creatine remains unknown, but at the very least grapefruit juice is a good source of sugar. It can't hurt to give it a try.

THIRD GENERATION

As would be expected the success of second generation creatine supplements opened the floodgates for research. The relationship between sugar and insulin was the first step, but newer substances have now come on the scene. Most third generation supplements owe their success to diabetes research. Taking actual insulin is one way to boosting insulin levels, but the trend now days is to look for substances that mimic insulin. The popularity of chromium and vanadyl supplements are two examples.

Lipoic acid is a substance that's getting a lot of press and promotion lately. Most of what we know about lipoic acid comes from research carried out in Europe, where physicians are using it to treat mild forms of diabetes. Mild being individuals who produce some insulin on their own, but not enough to adequately regulate blood sugar. Lipoic acid is to assist insulin in this role. Of course once creatine manufacturers heard of this wonderful new substance, they began adding it to their products.

First out of the blocks in this regard was MuscleTech of Canada. Their new product, Cell-Tech, contains 200 milligrams of lipoic acid per serving (in addition to the now almost mandatory sugar; which in Cell-Tech's case is dextrose). According to MuscleTech, Cell-Tech is up to 500 percent more effective than second generation creatine products. MuscleTech appears to be on to something, as most of the other big supplement manufacturers are now coming out with their own third generation creatine supplements.

THE LATEST RESEARCH

The following section summarizes some of the latest studies released since we wrote *Anabolic Primer*. Rather than bore you with details of how the experiments were carried out, we'll simply give you the results and how they apply to athletics.

AT THE HEART OF THE MATTER

With most research on creatine focusing on athlete's muscles, it's refreshing to see a study that looks at creatine's benefits to heart patients.

A recent European study gave heart patients (who had experienced congestive heart failure) five grams of creatine per day for five days. After the experiment concluded the patients were tested on a number of tasks including grip strength. The creatine-using group had stronger and more sustainable contractions than the control group. The researchers concluded that creatine supplementation holds great promise in helping heart patients regain physical strength and stamina.

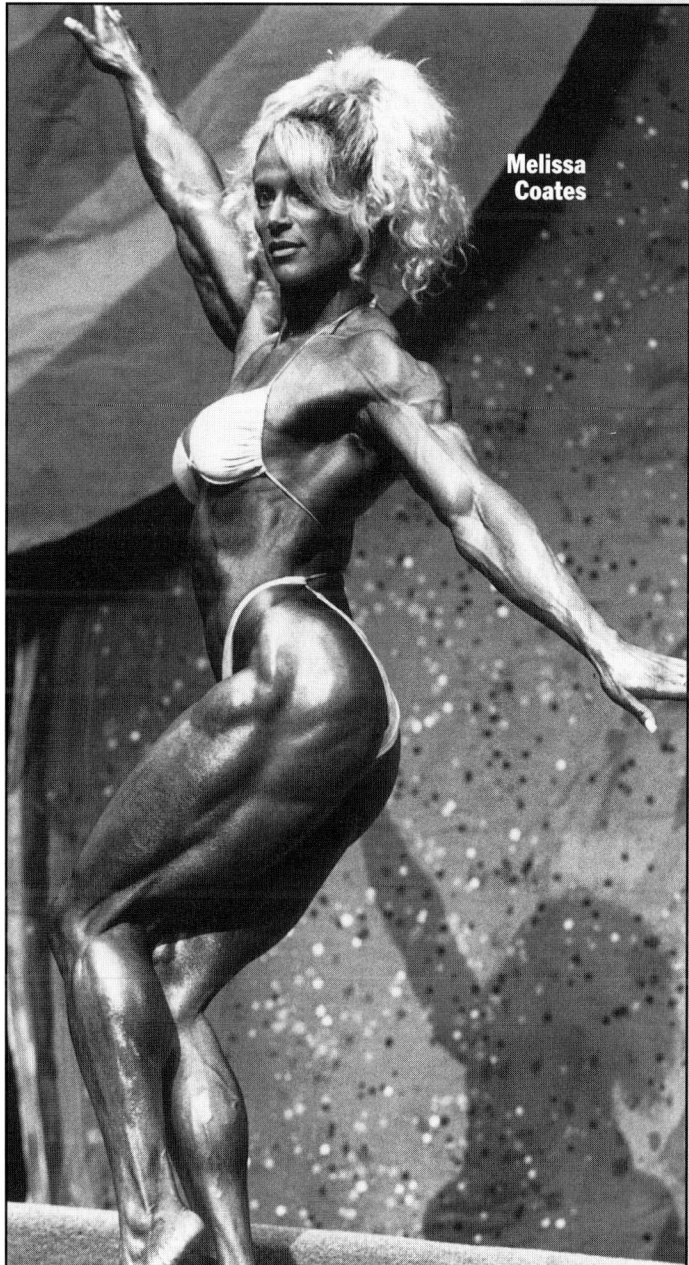

Melissa Coates

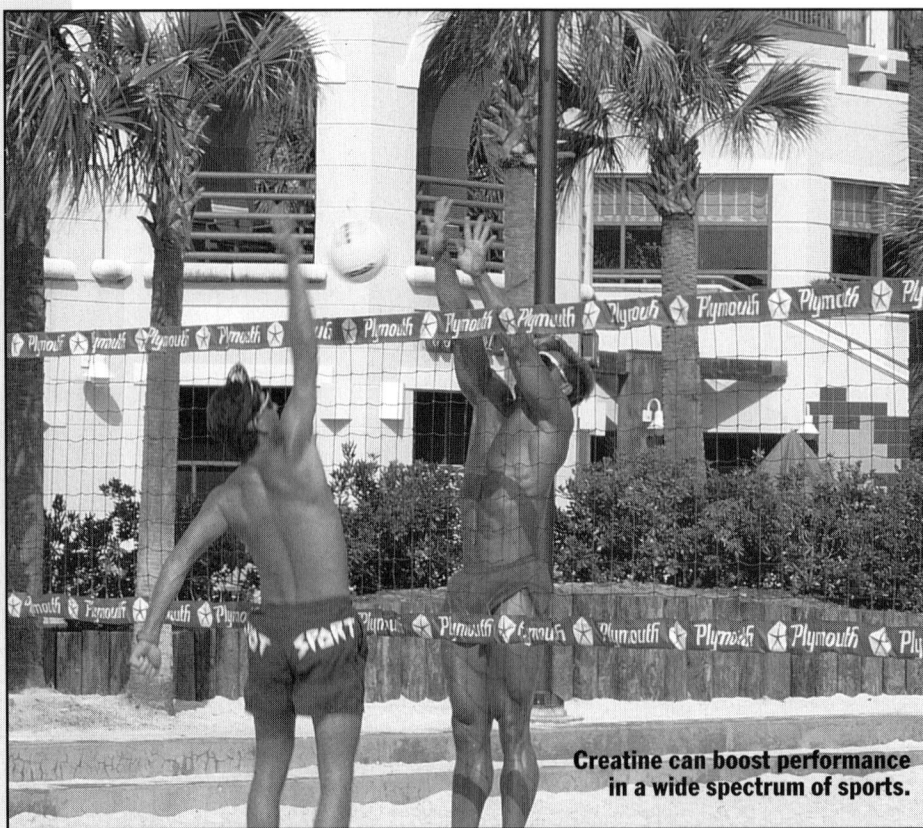

Creatine can boost performance in a wide spectrum of sports.

NOT JUST FOR BODYBUILDERS

Another study suggests that creatine is not just for athletes in anaerobic power sports. Researchers gave triathletes six grams of creatine per day, for five days. After administering a test that alternated between aerobic and anaerobic exercise, the researchers found that the creatine-using group showed less reduction in blood glucose than the control group. Creatine can play a role in boosting performance in a wide spectrum of sports.[2]

MORE EVIDENCE FOR ENDURANCE SPORTS

If you're not convinced yet, another study confirms creatine's role in aerobic sports. Instead of looking at athletes, researchers compared fast and slow twitch muscle fibers following creatine supplementation. Both muscle types had elevated levels of phosphocreatine. They also discovered elevated levels of the aerobic enzyme citrate synthase. Such findings add further evidence that athletes in aerobic sports can benefit from regular supplementation with creatine.[3]

FOR FAT LOSS TOO

Just when we thought all the effects of creatine were known, along comes a study in the *International Journal of Sports Nutrition* that suggests creatine can speed fat loss. Researchers found that men given 20 grams a day, for two weeks, had a higher resting metabolic rate than control groups. Such results will come as good news to bodybuilders getting ready for a contest. Not only will creatine supplementation keep energy levels high, but it may also play a role in fat loss.[4]

"We have found no significant side effects from moderate use of creatine. There are hundreds of thousands of creatine users who experience no side effects."

– Dr. Ray Sahelian, author of *Creatine Nature's Muscle Builder*, commenting on the media's over-reaction to the deaths of three college wrestlers who happened to be using creatine.

USING CREATINE

Most readers are probably familiar with how to use creatine supplements. But for those using the supplement for the first time, here are a few tips. First of all despite the great appeal don't fall for cheaper products at ridiculously low prices. In more cases than not you're being ripped off big time. Stick with the big names like TwinLab, MuscleTech, EAS and Formula One.

Start out by taking a small amount – say in the two to three gram range. Side effects are rare, but it's better to find out you can't tolerate creatine with small dosages rather than large.

Load for five to seven days on 20 to 30 grams. The best way to do this is to take five grams, five or six times daily, rather than 25 to 30 grams all at once. Trust us, it's a lot easier on your digestive system. The purpose of loading is to top your muscles to the max. After a week you can switch to a maintenance dosage of five to 10 grams.

Finally, to prevent tolerance (the point where the body produces a diminished response to a given substance) we suggest cycling four to six weeks on, and two to three weeks off. This way the supplement should always give you good results.

SIDE EFFECTS

We really had no intention of including a side effects' section on creatine as the supplement is one of the safest out there. But a few media stories have changed our thinking and we feel obligated to respond.

In many cases the media treat supplements the way they treat Hollywood celebrities. First they build them up, and then they latch on to the smallest negative detail, blow it out of proportion and ruin lives. Over the last year creatine has faced a similar barrage. Initial stories called it the greatest thing since sliced bread. Now it's labeled a killer!

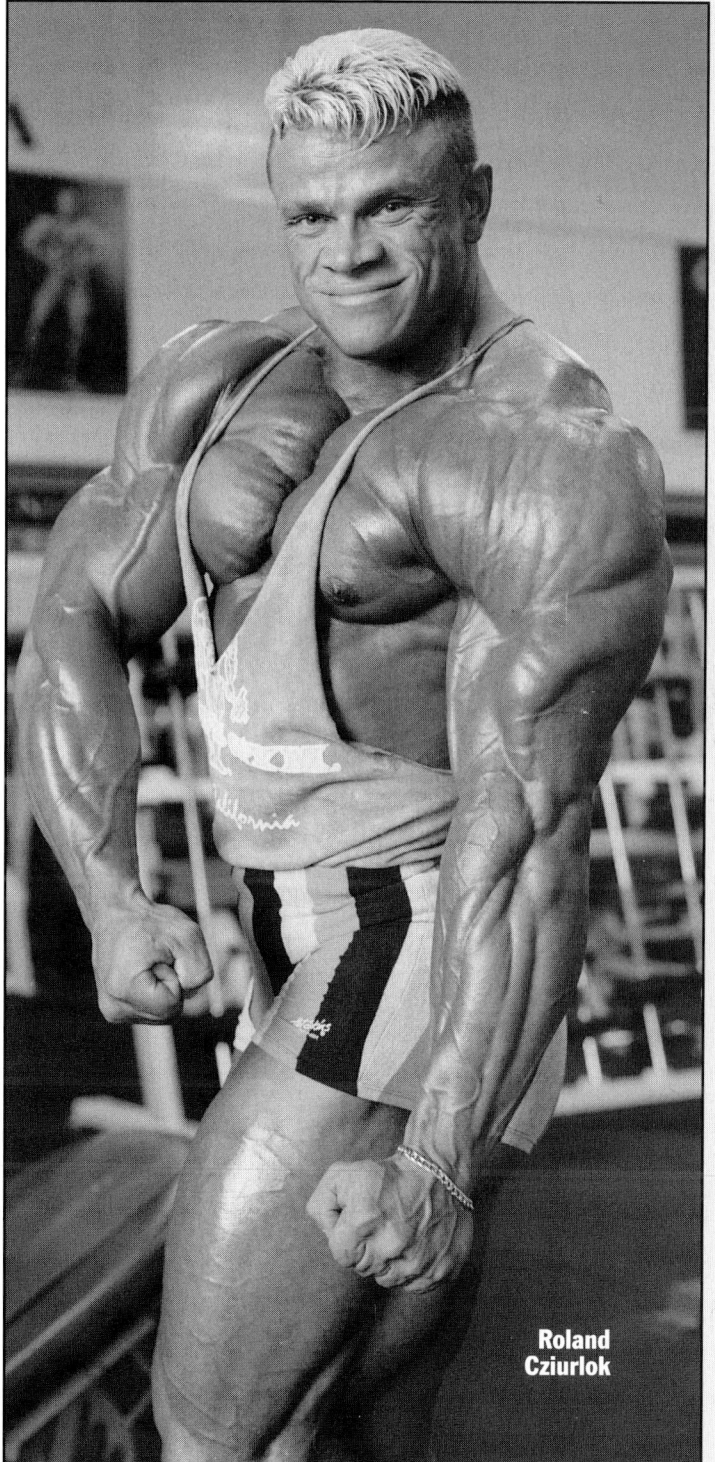

Roland Cziurlok

In the fall of 1997, three college wrestlers tragically died after trying to lose weight for a competition. This situation was no different than many others, as all too many athletes have died in the pursuit of achieving a desired physique. Unfortunately the media picked up on their creatine use and tried to make it sound as if the supplement killed them. The fact that the individuals were using other means to lose weight (poor eating, dehydration and, while no proof, possibly diuretics) was never mentioned. One of the athletes was attempting to lose 12 pounds by riding an exercise bike for two hours in a 92-degree room while wearing a rubber suit! Even after a few inquisitive journalists got to the heart of the mater, it was never reported with the same vigor as the original story.

For those new to creatine supplementation, let us state that creatine is one of the safest supplements you could ever use. The only side effects reported are a slight nausea and dehydration. Even then the problem is usually overdosing. Take five to 10 grams a day with plenty of water and you should have no problems. Don't let paranoid segments of the media frighten you away from one of the greatest athletic supplements ever produced.

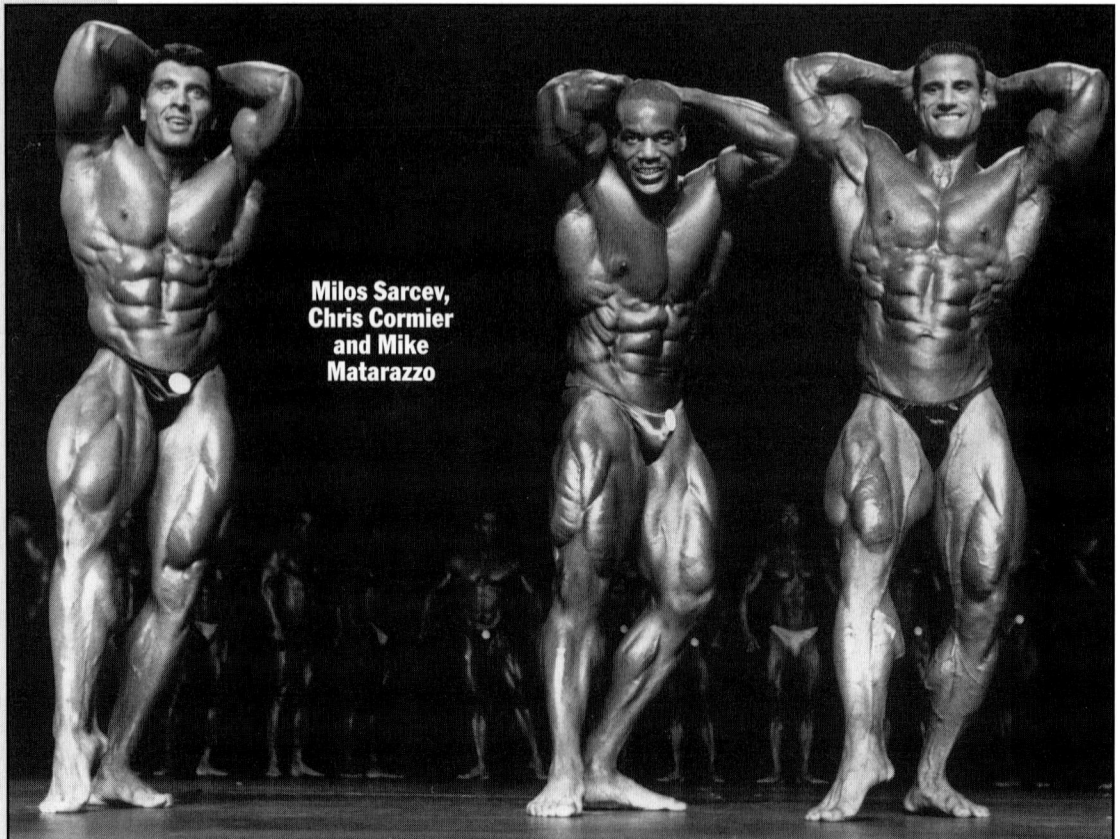

Milos Sarcev, Chris Cormier and Mike Matarazzo

References

1) Andrews, R, et al. The effect of dietary creatine supplementation on skeletal muscle metabolism in congestive heart failure. *European Heart Journal*, 19:617-622, 1998.
2) Engelhart, M, et al., Creatine supplementation in endurance sports. *Medicine and Science in Sports and Exercise*. 30:1123-1129, 1998.
3) Brannon, TA, et al. Effects of creatine loading and training on running performance and biochemical properties of rat skeletal muscle. *Medicine and Science in Sports and Exercise*, 29:489-495, 1997.
4) Arciero, RJ, Hannibal, NS, et al. Effects of creatine supplementation and weight training on resting metabolic rate and 1-RM in college-aged athletes. *International Journal of Sports Nutrition*, 8:199, 1998.
5) Putting the Squeeze on Grapefruit Juice. *Science News*, 153, 295, 1998.

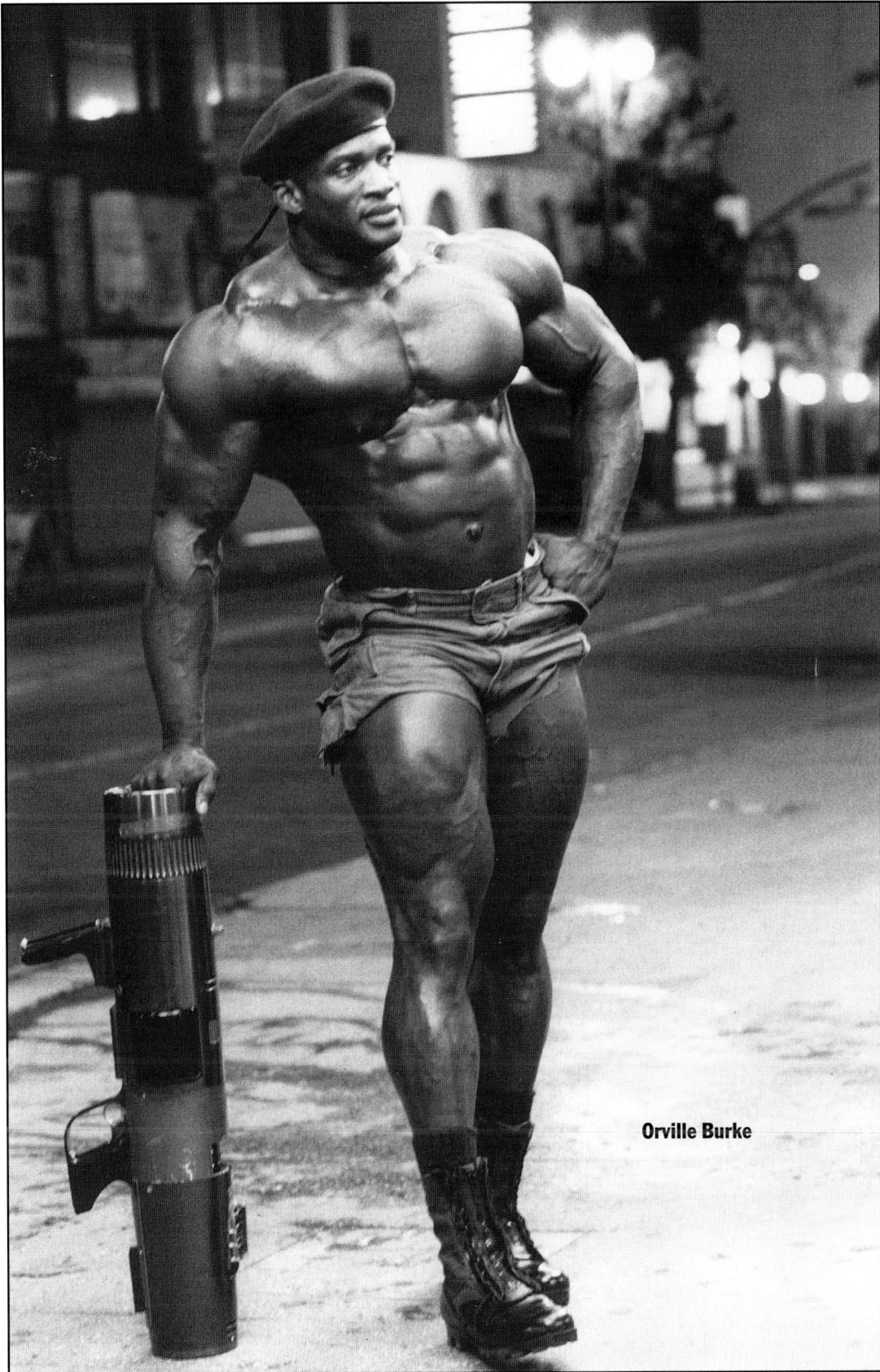

Orville Burke

CHAPTER THREE

Narcotic Analgesics

THE WALLY PIPP SYNDROME

Wally Pipp was the New York Yankees first baseman from 1915 to 1925. After developing a headache he was replaced by a relative unknown named Lou Gehrig. Pipp never again started in a game as first baseman for the Yankees; while Gehrig, who often played in pain, went on to immortality. If nothing else many athletes continue competing despite injury and pain, because their absence may lead to the discovery of an understudy or replacement. Competitive bodybuilders are all to familiar with contestants who can barely stand, but insist on going on stage when, in reality, their best option would be a hospital emergency room. Often the motivating fear is that a lower-ranked competitor might steal the spotlight. Let's face it, every year a whole new crop of bodybuilders qualify for pro level. Each with the mentality of a shark in a feeding frenzy – win at any cost.

The use of local analgesics is quite common in bodybuilding circles. Combinations of stimulants and painkillers were particularly popular among Olympic athletes in the 60s. One world record holder combined Darvon (a narcotic used to control skeletal pain and calm nerves) with methamphetamine (speed).[3]

"I was in absolute agony! I'd torn all the muscles in my lower back doing a poorly planned lift (I was showing off). It was an old injury, and it was back with a vengeance. I could barely walk. When I got to the hospital, the doctor examined me and ordered an injection of Demerol. The nurse gave me my shot in the butt, and a few minutes later, I was swept by a wave of nausea. The nurse reassured me, saying that the injection also included Gravol. Then it happened. My head floated off to my right. I could actually feel it, drifting just to the right of my shoulder. The pain totally disappeared, and the buzz kicked in. Euphoria is an understatement. A friend of mine pushed my wheelchair to the pharmacy, to pick up my prescription for painkillers. By the time we got to the pharmacy, I was having conversations with strangers (as I later learned, both real and imagined). I was very pleasant and managed to entertain the pharmacist and his staff. The rest of the afternoon is a complete blank, but I remember coming to my senses as the drug wore off. I can still remember the sensation of absolute inner peace, joy and harmony

"I think it's an incredibly tough position for everybody involved. I believe the doctors are trying to do their best, and the players are trying to do their best. But given the circumstances under which these decisions are made – mistakes happen."
– Bill Walton, basketball player, explaining his decision to accept injections of local anesthetics in the 1978 NBA playoff.

with the world around me. If you want a chemical definition of love, this is the closest you'll ever come to it. I could definitely train on it, but it would have to be a much lower dosage. I'd probably still get hooked. Definitely keep this stuff under lock-and-key!"
– An amateur bodybuilder relating his personal experience with the narcotic analgesic, Demerol.

WHAT THEY ARE

Any compound derived from opium poppy alkaloids (or any synthetic drugs with similar pharmacologic properties) are called narcotics or opiates. These drugs typically produce sedation (hypnosis) and analgesia, while reducing fear and anxiety. Morphine sulfate is the standard narcotic by which all others are measured. Narcotic effects are produced by stimulating opiate receptors in the brain (limbic system, thalamus and the hypothalamus). These receptors are organized into five classes:

Mu – Found in the pain-regulating areas of the brain. They contribute to the following actions: analgesia, euphoria, hypothermic, physical dependence and respiratory depression.

Kappa – Found in the spinal cord and cerebral cortex. They contribute to the following actions: miosis, sedation and analgesia.

Sigma – Possibly responsible for hallucinations and mydriatic effects.

Delta – Effects are unknown.

Epsilon – Effects are unknown.[1]

Among other things narcotic analgesics may produce euphoria and feelings of invincibility. They increase the pain threshold, such that the user may fail to recognize injury. Thus an injured bodybuilder could continue to workout, turning a mild problem into a serious one. These drugs are addictive and if used improperly can cause respiratory problems and even death. An effective dose that can be tolerated by habitual users can become lethal if consumed with alcohol (a non-bodybuilder example is the late rock singer, Janis Joplin). The following are narcotic analgesics that have been used as performance enhancing drugs. They are all banned by the IOC.[2]

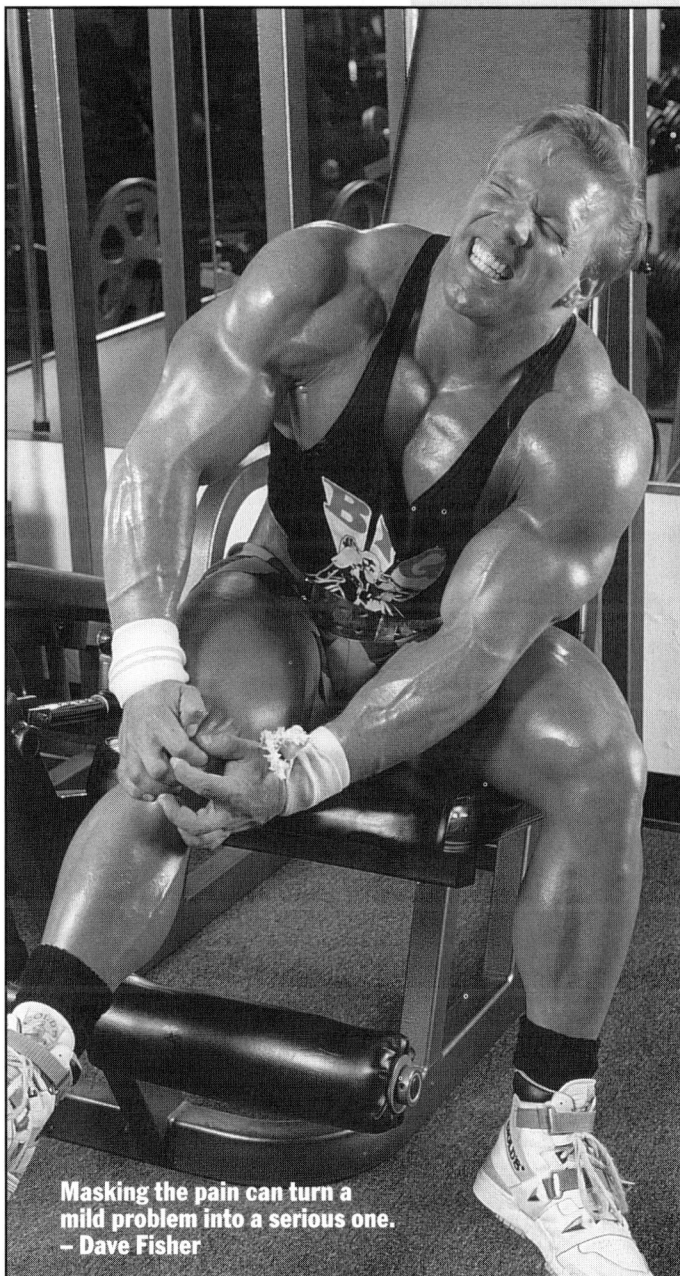

Masking the pain can turn a mild problem into a serious one.
– Dave Fisher

Roland Cziurlok

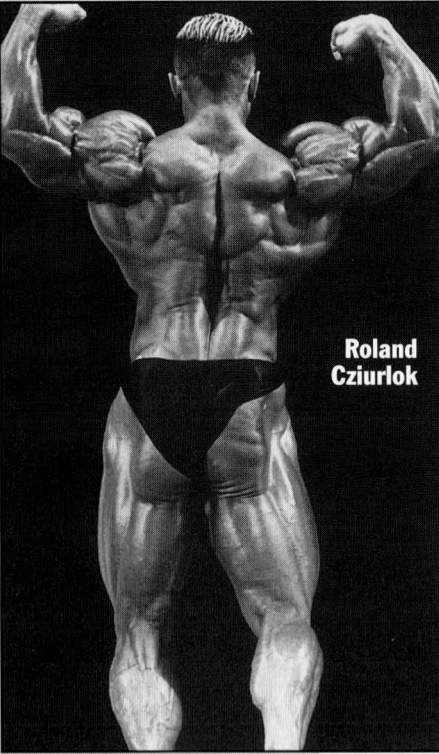

Trade Name: Nubain
Generic Name: Nalbuphine HCL
Dosage: 10 mg/70 kg, i.m., s.c. or i.v. every 3 to 6 hours
A maximum single dose of 20mg, and a maximum total daily dose of 160 mg

Comments: Nalbuphine is a synthetic, narcotic, agonist-antagonist analgesic; chemically related to the narcotic oxymorphone and the narcotic antagonist naloxone. This drug is used for moderate to severe pain. Possible side effects include: habit formation, sedation, clammy skin, nausea, vomiting, vertigo, dry mouth, headache, blurred vision, impaired speech, itching, cramps, dyspepsia, bitter taste, hypertension, hypotension, tachycardia, bradycardia, nervousness, crying, depression, hallucinations, euphoria, dysphoria, hostility and unusual dreams.[3]

Trade Names: Talwin Injection, Talwin Tablets
Generic Names: Pentazocine Lactate, Pentazocine HCL
Dosage: For Pentazocine Lactate, 30 mg i.m., s.c., or i.v., every 3 to 4 hours as needed, total daily maximum dose of 360 mg
For Pentazocine HCL, 50 to 100 mg orally with food, every 4 hours as needed

Comments: Pentazocine is a member of the benzazocine series of synthetic benzomorphans. It produces both analgesic (agonist) and narcotic antagonist effects. A dose of 30 milligrams injected is approximately equal in analgesic activity to 10 milligrams of morphine or 75 to 100 milligrams of meperidine. Fifty milligrams of pentazocine taken orally is about the same in analgesic activity as 60 milligrams of codeine. Among the potential side effects are: habit formation, physical and mental impairment (precluding the operation of heavy machinery and driving) and urinary retention.

Trade Names: Demerol and Mepergan
Generic Name: Meperidine HCL
Dosage: 50 to 150 mg orally (least effective), s.c. or i.m., every 3 to 4 hours as needed.

Comments: This narcotic analgesic has multiple actions similar to those of morphine; the most prominent involves the CNS and organs composed of smooth muscle. The main actions of therapeutic value are sedation and analgesia. On a milligram basis, meperidine has one-tenth the strength of morphine. Meperidine's onset of action is more rapid than that of morphine, but has a shorter duration. Meperidine can cause nausea, and is usually given with dimenhydrate (Gravol). Other side effects include: euphoria, lightheadedness, vertigo, sedation and sweating. Other possible serious side effects (potentially fatal ones) include: respiratory depression, respiratory arrest, circulatory depression and cardiac arrest. Drug interactions can lead to respiratory depression, hypotension, profound sedation and coma. The following drugs can interact with meperidine: CNS depressants (including alcohol, tricyclic antidepressants, sedative-hypnotics (including the barbiturates), tranquilizers, phenothiazines, other narcotic analgesics and general anesthetics.[3]

Trade Names: Hycodan, Tussionex ,
  Vicodin, Hycomine, Hycomine-S
Generic Names: Hydrocodone Bitartrate, Hydrocodone Compound
Dosage: For Hydrocone Bitartrate (first 3 trade names),
  5 mg (1 tablet or 1 ml) orally, every 4 hours, with food,
  not to exceed 30 mg within 24 hours; maximum single dose of 15 mg
  For Hydrocodone Compound, Hycomine,
  5 mg (5 ml) orally, every 4 hours with food, not to exceed
  30 mg within 24 hours; maximum single dose of 15 mg
  For Hydrocodone Compound, Hycomine-S,
  5 mg (10 ml) orally, every 4 hours, with food, not to
  exceed 30 mg within 24 hours; maximum single dose of 10 mg.

Comments: Hydrocodone is an antitussive agent that is two to eight times as potent as codeine. At equi-effective doses, hydrocodone has a greater sedative action than codeine. The exact mechanism of action is unknown, but hydrocodone is believed to directly depress the cough centre. Therapeutic doses can also produce an analgesic effect. It is usually used to control a severe cough. Among the many possible side effects are: respiratory depression, addiction, nausea, vomiting, urinary retention, impairment of physical and mental performance, mood changes and blurred vision. The hydrocodone compound also includes phenylephrine (which is contraindicated in individuals with hyperthyroidism), heart disease, diabetes and hypertension. Phenylephrine can have negative inter-actions with certain drugs, so the following should be avoided: methlydopa, monoamine oxidase (MAO) inhibitors, beta-blockers and indomethacin.[3]

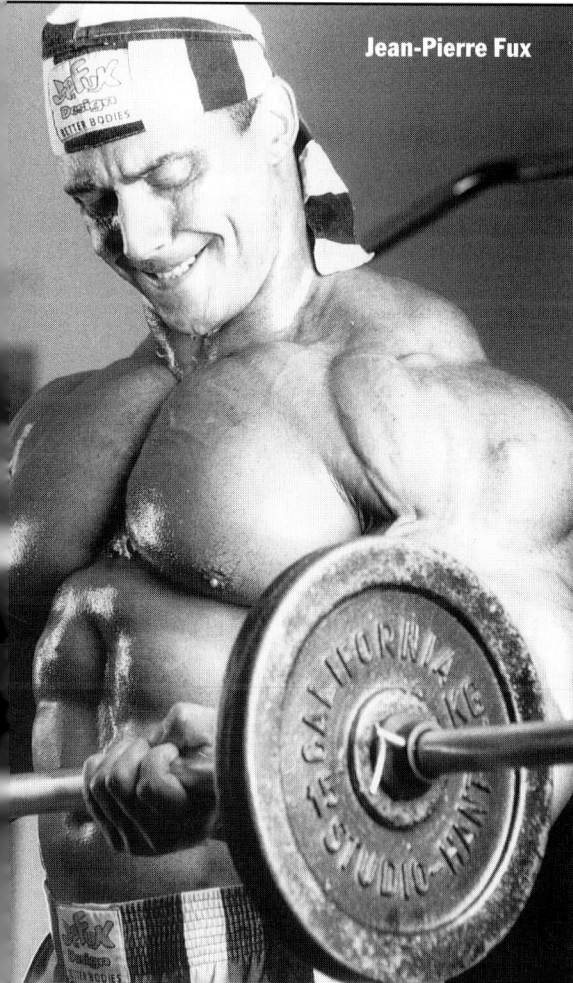

Jean-Pierre Fux

Trade Names: Percodan,
  Percodan-Demi, Tylox
Generic Name: Oxycodone
  HCL-ASA
Dosage: Percodan Tablet
  (5 mg oxydocone, 325 mg ASA)
  every 6 hours
  1 to 2 Percodan-Demi Tablets
  (2.5mg oxydocone, 325 ASA)
  every 6 hours

Comments: Oxycodone is a semisyn-thetic narcotic analgesic with actions similar to morphine, the most prominent of which involve the CNS and organs that are composed of smooth muscle. Oxycodone's therapeutic values are its analgesic and sedative actions. ASA (aspirin) is a non-narcotic, anti-inflam-matory and antipyretic analgesic. This drug is used to treat mild to moderately

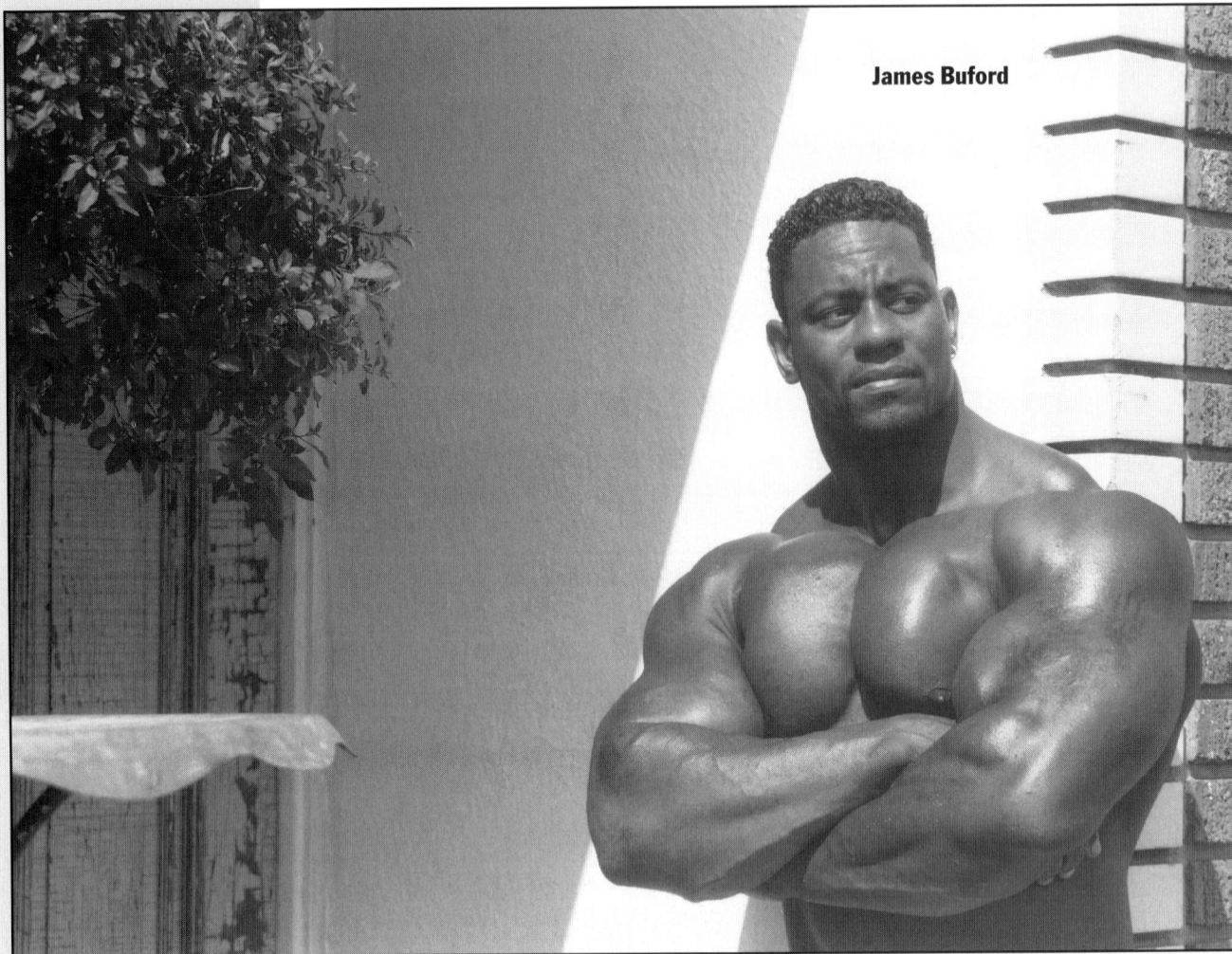

James Buford

severe pain, including conditions accompanied by inflammation and/or fever. It is habit forming and should not be used while operating heavy machinery or driving. The possible side effects include: lightheadedness, nausea, vertigo, constipation, dysphoria, euphoria, pruritis and vomiting. The following drugs can interact with oxycodone: CNS depressants (including alcohol), sedative hypnotics, other narcotic analgesics, phenothiazines, tricyclic antidepressants, monoamine oxidase inhibitors, other tranquilizers and general anesthetics.[3]

Trade Name: Numorphan
Generic Name: Oxymorphone HCL
Dosage: 1 to 1.5 mg s.c. or i.m., repeat every 4 to 6 hours as needed
5 mg rectal suppository, repeat every 4 to 6 hours as needed

Comments: This drug is a potent narcotic analgesic. An injection of 1 milligram is equivalent to 10 milligrams of morphine sulfate. Injected oxymorphone has a rapid onset, and the effects can be felt within five to 10 minutes. The analgesic effect will last around three to six hours. This drug can be habit forming, and may cause the following side effects: mild sedation, respiratory depression, headache, nausea, vomiting, lightheadedness, itching and dysphoria.[3]

> Trade Names: Dilaudid, Dilaudid Sterile Powder,
> Dilaudid-HP Parenteral
> Generic Name: Hydromorphone HCL
> (A hydrogenated ketone of morphine)
> Dosage: 2 to 4 mg orally, every 4 to 6 hours as required,
> or 2 mg s.c. or i.m., every 4 to 6 hours
> Severe pain can be controlled by 3 to 4 mg, every 4 to 6 hours
> 3 mg rectal suppositories provide long-lasting relief,
> which is useful at night

Comments: This drug has potent analgesic and antitussive properties. The drug will begin to exert its effect about 15 minutes after injection, and the analgesic effect should last about five hours. Oral doses take about 30 minutes to exert an effect. Hydromorphone HCL is eight times more powerful than morphine on a milligram basis. It has numerous possible side effects including: nausea, constipation and stupor. It can cause drug dependence, and is contraindicated for anyone with asthma or other respiratory problems. An overdose can lead to respiratory failure and death. Additive depressant effects can be produced if Hydromorphone HCL is taken with other CNS depressants including: sedatives, general anesthetics, phenothiazines, tranquilizers and alcohol.[3]

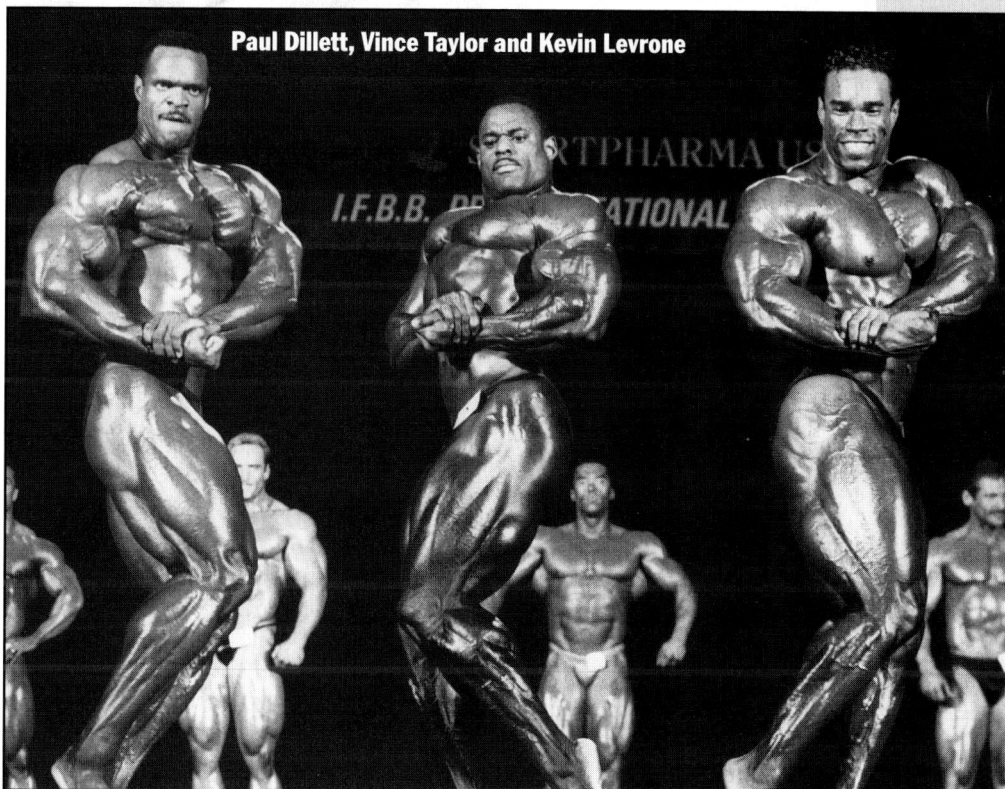

Paul Dillett, Vince Taylor and Kevin Levrone

References

1) Tobin, T. *Drugs and the Performance Horse*, Charles C. Thomas, Publisher, Springfield, Illinois, 1981.
2) United States Olympic Committee. Narcotic Analgesics, *Drug Control Education*, http://www.olympic-usa.org/inside/in 1_3_7_2.html.
3) Krogh, C (chief ed.). *CPS, Compendium of Pharmaceuticals and Specialties*, 30th edition, Canadian Pharmaceutical Association, Ottawa, 1995.

CHAPTER FOUR

Fat Loss

"Non-fat diets will make you fat in the long run. Over the years we have grown to think of fat as our enemy, when it's our friend."

– Mia Finnegan, top fitness competitor responding to an *Oxygen* reader's question about fat.

BETA AGONISTS

In their never-ending quest to shed bodyfat, bodybuilders and other athletes have been known to try just about any substance that comes along. Beta agonists are one of the most popular, but as with any drug, precautions must be taken.

Beta agoinsts stimulate special receptors throughout the body called beta-receptors. Molecular biologists have classified the known receptor sites throughout the body based on characteristics including location and mechanism of action. There are even differences within receptor types. For example, beta-receptors fall into at least three subtypes (beta 1, 2 and 3), and odds are more will be discovered.

WHY BETA AGONISTS?

Beta agonists are very efficient at reducing bodyfat and enhancing lean tissue deposition. The agents used are relatively specific for the beta-2 receptor. These agents work by decreasing lipogenesis (fat formation) and enhancing lipolysis (fat breakdown) in adipose (fat) tissue. In skeletal muscles, their primary effect is to reduce the rate of protein degradation. The beta-receptor is subject to regulation by other hormones and, not surprisingly, beta-agonists can influence the circulatory concentrations of several endogenous hormones.[2]

Beta agonists have the properties of both hormones and neurotransmitters (of the sympathetic system). The sympathetic nervous system is part of the autonomous nervous system. Its major activities include: the stimulation of cardiac functions (force and frequency), the tone of blood vessels, the gut and bronchial muscles and metabolic system: glycogenolysis, sugar breakdown, and lipolysis, fat breakdown. In general, the sympathetic system is activated during high intensity physical activity. The main neurotransmitter for this system is noradrenalin, a catecholamine produced from the amino acid tyrosine. The adrenal glands produce both noradrenalin and adrenalin hormones. Their physiological functions include circulatory effects, the stimulation of glycogenolysis (glucose formation from stored glycogen) and lipolysis.

Beta agonists are close analogues of noradrenalin and adrenalin. The beta-1 receptor has a roughly equivalent affinity for the two hormones, while the beta-2 receptor exhibits a greater affinity for adrenalin. Beta-2 agonists are safer than beta-1 agonists, because beta-2 agonists are less likely to affect the heart (although it's still a risk for heart patients to use them).

EXAMPLES OF COMMONLY USED BETA AGOINSTS

Trade Names: Spiropent, Ventolase, Ventapulmin, Prontovent, Oxyflux, Novegam, Monores, Contraspasmina, Contrasmina, Clenbuter.Pharmachim, Clenasma, Cesbron, Broncoterol, Broncodil
Generic Name: Clenbuterol
Dosage: 2 tablets (10 mcg or 20 mcg strength) twice a day, 2 days on, 2 days off, for 2 weeks, or 80 to 140 mcg/day, in split doses, 2 weeks on and 2 weeks off

Comments: This drug stimulates the beta-2 and beta-3 receptors in fat and muscle tissue. While it has proven to be anabolic in livestock, the same effects are not always seen in humans. One theory is that we don't have enough beta-3 receptors (cattle have an abundance). The main value of this drug is its ability to act as a fat burner through thermogenesis. Every degree that it raises body temperature, an additional five percent of maintenance calories will be burned. To counteract this, the body cuts down on thyroid hormone production and begins down regulation of the receptors. This is why experts believe you only have a limited time in which clenbuterol can be effective. However, the following appears to refute this position. It is possible for clenbuterol to be used as a long-term diet drug. A medical student in Mexico reported that he took two tablets in the morning and two at noon, Monday to Friday, for 12 months. He took them for breathing problems due to the poor air quality in Guadalajara. When he began taking clenbuterol, he was 250 pounds at 36 percent bodyfat. After a year he was 220 pounds, at 11 percent bodyfat. In other words, a loss of 75 pounds of bodyfat. His training regimen was one to one and a half hours, Monday to Saturday.[5]

There is some controversy over the best method to take clenbuterol. A cycling theory of two days on and two days off is suggested by *MuscleMedia* publisher, Bill Phillips. It is based on the idea that periodically decreasing the amount of drug would reduce receptor desensitization. The problem with this idea is the half-life of clenbuterol. It is metabolized by biphasic elimination, the rapid phase lasting 10 hours, and the slow phase lasting several days. So even after two days off, the body still has over 50 percent of the

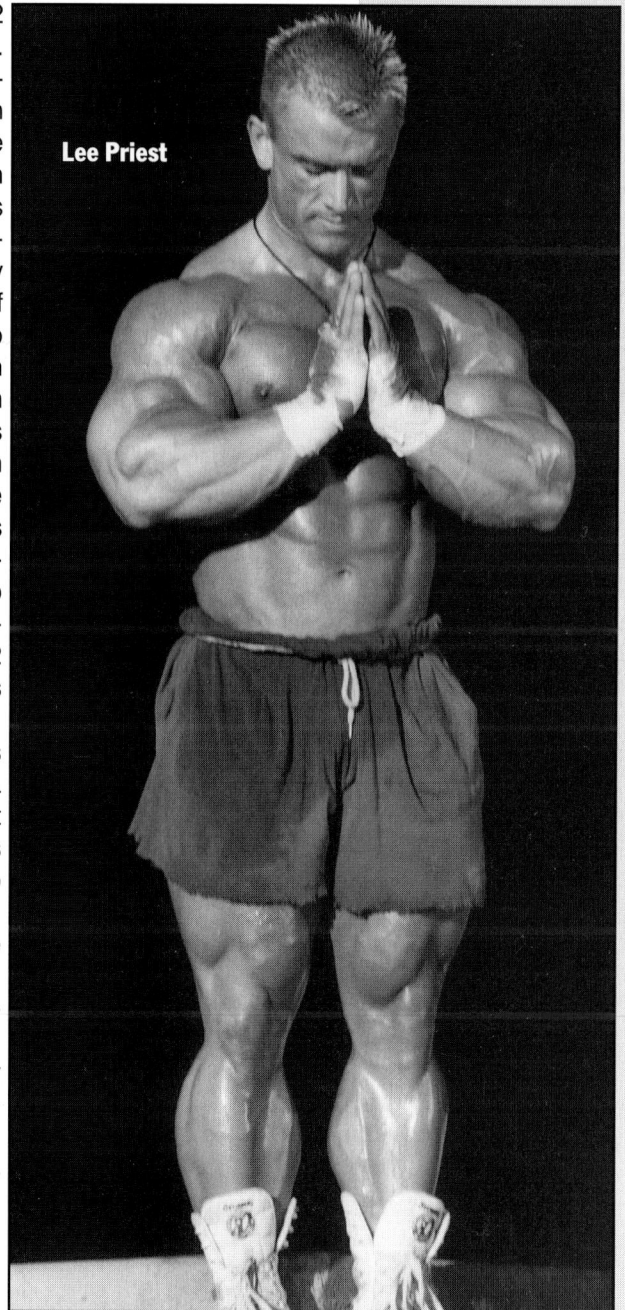

Lee Priest

previous clenbuterol dosage in active form. The two weeks on and two weeks off method has the disadvantage of leaving the user with low energy levels. Of course ephedrine might be an option for restoring energy levels during the two weeks off clenbuterol.[6] But as a word of caution you are now starting to fall into the trap of using one drug to assist another drug. Before long a state of polypharmacology exists. You're now taking multiple drugs to modify your lifestyle. We are going to leave the moral implications of this to you, the reader. But from a physiological point of view the more drugs you use, and the longer you stay on them, the greater the risk of side effects.

OTHER EXAMPLES OF BETA AGONISTS

Trade Names: Albuterol, Ventolin Inhaler, Proventil Inhaler
Generic Name: Salbutamol

Trade Name: Combivent
Generic Name: Salbutamol/Ipratropium

Trade Name: Brethaire
Generic Name: Terbutaline

Trade Name: Serevent
Generic Name: Salmeterol

Trade Names: Isuprel, Norisodrine, Metihaler-ISO
Generic Name: Isoproterenol

Trade Names: Alupent, Metaprel
Generic Name: Metaproterenol

Generic Name: Fenoterol

Generic Name: Isoxuperine

Generic Name: Pirbuterol

Generic Name: Cimaterol (One part-per-million (ppm) in the diet results in a higher muscle content of the carcass and reduced fat deposition; the final result being in a way a repartition of meat and fat tissues in favor of a higher meat content.[3])

EFFECTS ON PROSTAGLANDINS

Prostaglandins are hormone-like substances that play a role in modulating just about every metabolic activity in the human body. At one time bio-chemists only gave them a casual glance, but now they're the focus of a great deal of research. One role they play is in the control of protein synthesis and degradation. There is research to suggest that beta agonists may interfere with the synthesis of some of the prostaglandins, which have been associated with the control of muscle protein breakdown.[2] For bodybuilders this may explain why beta agonists are so valuable. In effect they are muscle sparing and allow fat to be lost without sacrificing muscle tissue.

TOO MUCH OF A GOOD THING?

One aspect that should not be underestimated is the phenomenon of receptor down-regulation and desensitization. Continued exposure of a receptor to a drug leads to a blunted response. This diminishing effect is accompanied by a decrease in the affinity of the drug's receptors (a process called uncoupling), followed by a decrease in the density (the number of receptors per unit area) of the receptor (a process known as down-regulation). Both processes can influence the effectiveness of a given drug, to cause what is known as tolerance. One potential theory is that in some cells, receptor molecules might, upon stimulation, be taken up by the cell's cytosol and then metabolized intracellularly. It appears that the rate – but probably not the level – of down-regulation (receptor-loss) is determined by each cells unique qualities.[6]

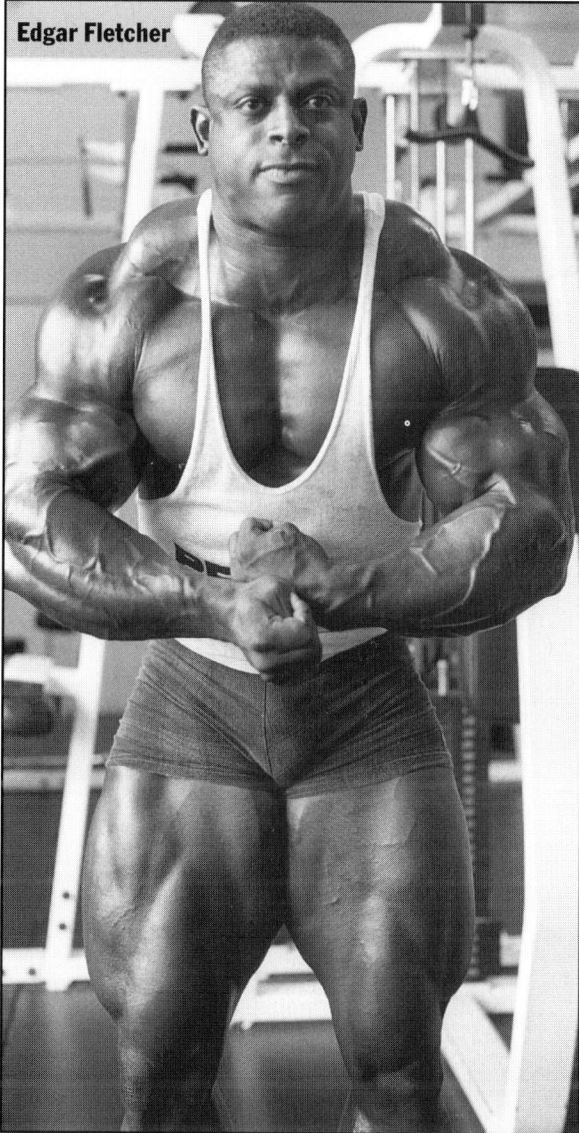

Edgar Fletcher

BETA-3 AGONISTS, FUTURE FAT BURNERS?

It could be that many of today's best-known diet drugs and cycles might soon become a thing of the past. There is plenty of evidence to demonstrate the role of beta-2 receptors in thermogenesis. But what about drugs that only select beta-3 receptors? They could very well be the drugs of the future.

Researchers at the University of Ottawa have shown that rats given beta-3 agonists increased their resting metabolic rates by 40 to 45 percent. The researchers found that the effect was produced by increasing thermogenesis in white and brown fat deposits.[15]

The beta-3 receptor is located on the surface of adipocytes (fat cells). Upon exposure, norepinephrine (noradrenalin) binds to beta-3 receptors, causing cyclic AMP (found in the fat cells) to stimulate the breakdown of fat stored within the cell. This results in the spilling of free fatty acids (FFAs) into the blood. FFAs from white adipose go to the liver, and those from brown adipose are burned. Brown adipose contains a fair number of beta-3 receptors. Therefore the beta-3 receptor plays a role in regulating the body's metabolic rate through the process of thermogenesis.

Of course, there are cons to this form of treatment. The beta-3 receptor is found on other organs, and their unintended stimulation might result in harmful side effects. Also, while some evidence suggests beta-3 agonists can stimulate white adipose tissue, the effect is primarily seen at brown adipose deposits – something humans have low amounts of. This raises the question, why focus on it? Still this is one area of research that should be watched closely in the near future.

The following are two examples of beta-3 agonists. The drugs are so new that they still don't have names.

DRUG: CL316,243
Comments: This is a prototypical beta-3 agonist that stimulates fat breakdown and thermogenesis in fat cells.

DRUG: L1739,574
Comments: This drug is more specific for the human beta-3 receptor. It has had good effects in Rhesus monkeys and has also been shown to increase the rate of fat breakdown and the metabolic rate.[7]

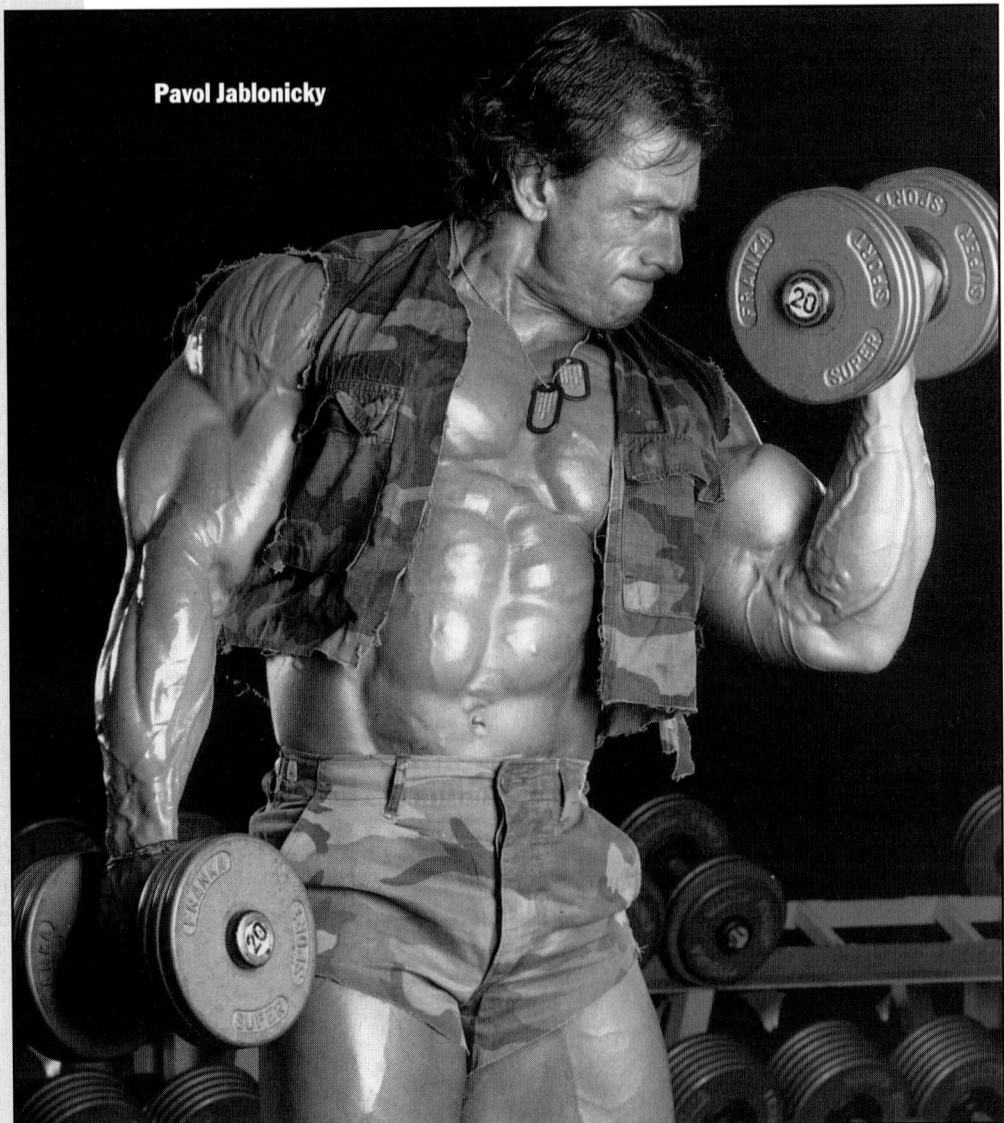

Pavol Jablonicky

L-CARNITINE

Later in this book we will look at a form of this substance that may increase testosterone levels (see Testosterone Precursors and Related Substances). For now we will briefly explore the potential of carnitine as a fat loss agent.

HOW IT WORKS

Carnitine is a substance that plays a major role in fat oxidation, by transporting fatty acids from the cytosol into the mitochondria of cells. The mitochondria are engine rooms in cells, being the chief energy producing organelle. Long chain fatty acid metabolism is heavily dependent on carnitine. When carnitine is deficient, fatty acid metabolism is impaired. In such cases, taking carnitine supplements improves fatty acid oxidation.[8] The question, however, is does carnitine increase fat burning in healthy individuals?

A ROLE IN ATHLETICS?

Manufacturers of carnitine supplements continuously promote the substance as a fat loss agent. In deficient people this is backed up by science, but not in healthy individuals. Numerous studies giving healthy subjects two to six grams of carnitine a day found no increase in fatty acid oxidation compared to control groups.[9, 10]

However, supplement manufacturers still promote carnitine to athletes in sports requiring fat loss – particularly those sports where weight classes exist (bodybuilding, wrestling and boxing). Besides the lack of evidence for fat loss in healthy individuals, there's little evidence to suggest athletes are deficient in carnitine, as opposed to other minerals like zinc and iron. Finally, studies with athletes megadosing on carnitine found that carnitine levels increased only by one to two percent.[11] Hardly enough to justify the risk and expense of carnitine supplementation.

CAFFEINE

Caffeine is one of the cheapest, yet effective over-the-counter drugs available. In fact, caffeine is so effective, the International Olympic Committee (IOC) has placed caffeine on its restricted drugs list (amounts more than 12 milligrams per liter of urine).

Athletes use caffeine for two reasons – fat loss and stimulation. As we are mainly concerned with fat loss, suffice to say caffeine is probably the world's most popular stimulant, and few households go without having it in one form or the other (coffee, tea and chocolate being the most popular).

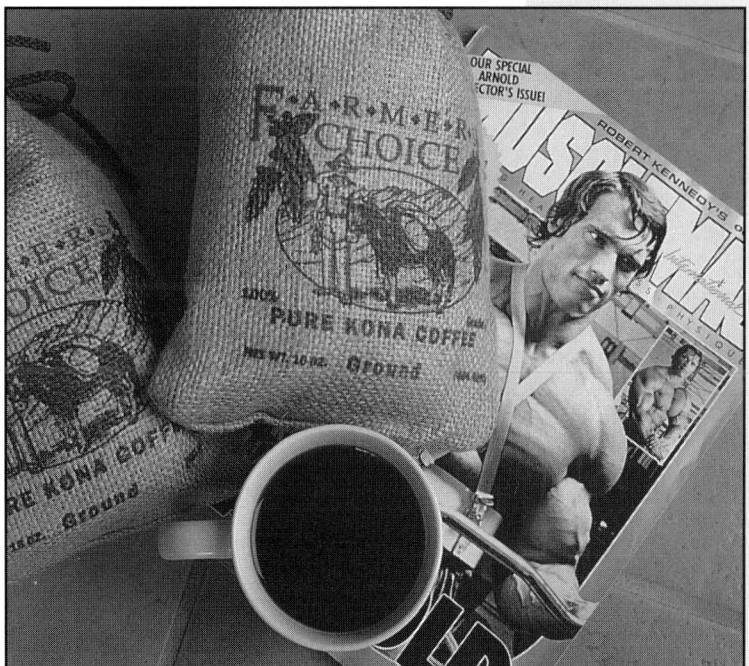

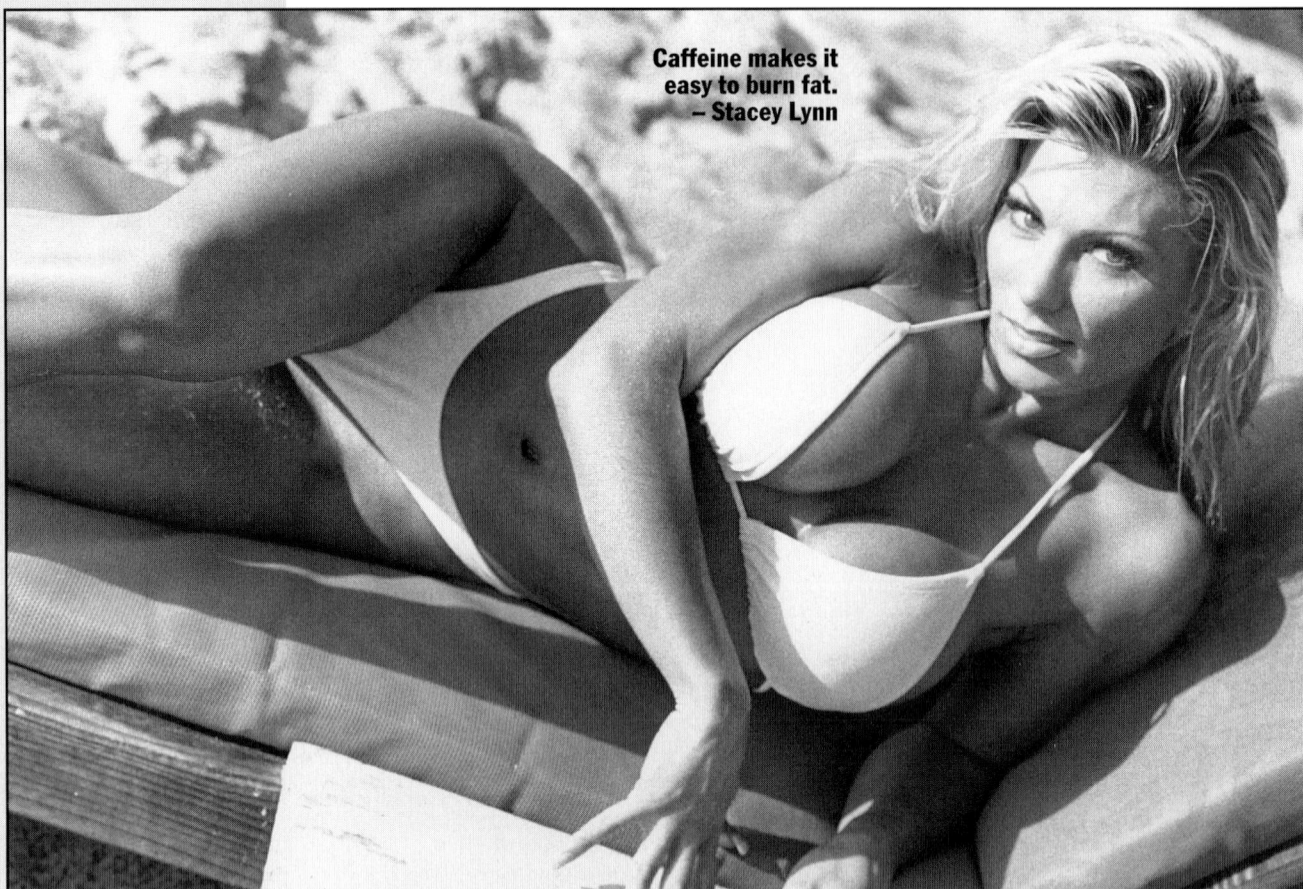

Caffeine makes it
easy to burn fat.
– Stacey Lynn

Besides stimulation, caffeine is also classified as a thermogenic drug. That is it slightly elevates body temperature, thus making fat stores easier to burn as a fuel source.[12, 13]

USING CAFFEINE

Among bodybuilders, the most popular way to take caffeine is to stack one cup of coffee (or 250 milligram equivalent), with 25 milligrams of ephedrine and one aspirin. These three drugs taken together produce what is called the synergistic effect. Each drug magnifies the effects of the other two.

Being a stimulant, those with heart problems should check first with their physician before using caffeine. A few users report a slight burning sensation or nausea after caffeine ingestion, but for the most part caffeine is safe. Like any drug the risk of side effects increases with dosage. A few studies have linked heart disease with heavy caffeine use, but the equivalent of one or two cups of coffee per day should not pose a serious health threat to most users.

HYDROXY CITRIC ACID – HCA

Hydroxy citric acid or HCA is in many respects similar to vitamins and mineral supplements. You could be taking it for years and not realize the benefits it's making to your health.

HCA is getting a lot of press these days not as a fat burning agent, but as a fat preventing agent. This is why most of the top supplement manufacturers combine it with fat burning substances like ephedrine. In a manner of speaking you get the best of both worlds – one substance to get rid of existing fat, while the other prevents the build up of new fat deposits.

Darrem Charles

HCA is the active ingredient found in the rinds of the fruit Garcinia cambogia. Studies with animals suggest it works in two manners. First, it has the ability to suppress appetite. We don't need to go into detail on how this would aid fat loss. The less excess calories taken in, the less potential for fat storage.

The second method of action involves a tad bit more biochemistry. HCA seems to have the ability to interfere with an enzyme called ATP-citrate lyase. Among other things this enzyme converts excess carbohydrate into fat. HCA blocks the actions of the enzyme, thus preventing such carbohydrate to fat conversion.[14]

Like many supplements discussed in this book, most of the information on HCA has come from animal studies. Still, this is a step in the right direction. The recommended dosage (based on anecdotal evidence we might add) is 750 to 1000 milligrams per day. Bodybuilders might want to give HCA a go during the precontest season. Don't expect anything dramatic, but it could give you that extra degree of hardness.

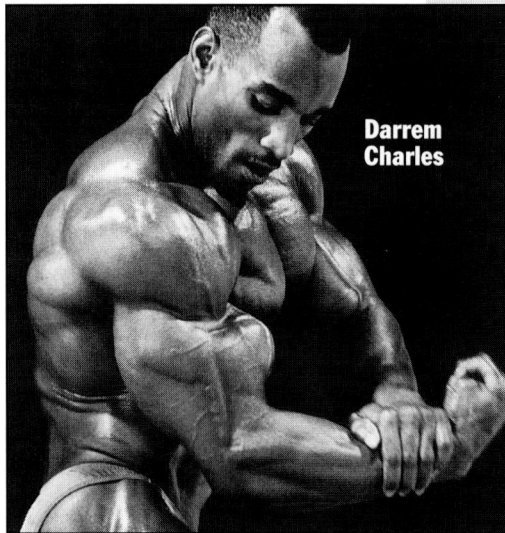

References
1) Timmerman, H. Beta-Adrenergics, Physiology, Pharmacology, Applications, Structures and Structure-Activity Relationships, in Hanrahan, J. (ed.): *Beta-Agonists and Their Effects On Animal Growth and Carcass Quality*, A Seminar in the CEC Program of Coordination of Research in Animal Husbandry, held in Brussels, 19 to 20 May, 1987, Elsevier Applied Science Publishers Ltd., Essex, 1987.
2) Buttery, P. and Dawson, J. The Mode Of Action Of Beta-Agonists As Manipulators of Carcass Composition, in Hanrahan, J. (ed.): *Beta-Agonists and Their Effects On Animal Growth and Carcass Quality*, A Seminar in the CEC Program of Coordination of Research in Animal Husbandry, held in Brussels, 19 to 20 May, 1987, Elsevier Applied Science Publishers Ltd., Essex, 1987.
3) Bekaert, H., Casteels, M. and Buysse, F. Effetcs of a Beta-agonist on Performance, Carcass and Meat Quality Of Growing-Finishing Pigs Of The Belgian Landrace, in Hanrahan, J. (ed.): *Beta-Agonists and Their Effects On Animal Growth and Carcass Quality*, A Seminar in the CEC Program of Coordination of Research in Animal Husbandry, held in Brussels, 19 to 20 May, 1987, Elsevier Applied Science Publishers Ltd., Essex, 1987.
4) United States Olympic Committee. Beta-2 Agonists, Drug Control Education, http://www.olympic-usa.org/inside/in_1_3_7_1.html.
5) *You Can Get Clenbuterol (Spiropent) Under Many Different Brand Names*, http://www.anabolicsteroids.com/clenbuterol.html. □
6) Clenbuterol. Drugs, *Absolute Truth Hardcore Bodybuilding*, http://members.tripod.com/~newguru/newclenbuterol.html.
7) Beta-3 Agonists: New Drugs for the Treatment of Obesity, http://PHARMINFO.COM/disease/diabetes/ADA97/ADA-7107.html
8) Stanley, C.A. New genetic defects in mitochondrial fatty acid oxidation and carnitine deficiency. *Adv Pediatr*, 34: 59-88, 1987.
9) Greig, C, et al. The effect of oral supplementation with L-carnitine on maximum and submaximum exercise capacity. *European Journal of Applied Physiology*, 56 (4), 457-460, 1987.
10) Trappe, S.W., et al. The effects of L-carnitine supplementation on performance during interval swimming. *International Journal of Sports Medicine*, 15 (4) 181-185, 1994.
11) Hultman, E., et al. Carnitine administration as a tool to modify energy metabolism during exercise, *European Journal of Applied Physiology*, 62 (6), 450, 1991.
12) Ivy, J.L., et al. Influence of caffeine and carbohydrate feedings on endurance performance. *Medicine and Science in Sports and Exercise*, 11 (1) 6-11, 1979.
13) Berglund, B., et al. Effects of caffeine ingestion on exercise performance at low and high altitudes in cross-country skiers. *International Journal of Sports Medicines*, 3 (4) 234-236, 1982.
14) Groff,J.L., et al. *Advanced Nutrition and Human Metabolism*, New York: West Publishing Co., 1995.
15) Ghorbam, M., et al., Hypertrophy of brown adipocytes in brown and white adipose tissue and reversal of diet induced obesity in rats treated with a beta-3 agonist. *Biochem Pharmacology*, 54, 121-131, 1997.

CHAPTER FIVE

Antibiotics and Their Use As Growth Promotants

The use of antibiotics in large-scale food production has been common place for the last 40 years. Animals fed a balanced diet, plus antibiotics, experience increased growth known as the Antibiotic Growth Effect (AGE). This effect has been the same over the years. An adaptogen-like effect is observed. Given a diet containing antibiotics, animals placed in a stressful environment actually grow more than animals in more a more pleasant climate. Further, very low levels of antibiotics are needed to obtain the AGE (10 grams per ton of feed). The exact mode of action is still not understood, but researchers agree that most of these drugs exert their effect within the gastrointestinal (GI) tract. The AGE is produced from various antibiotics of unrelated chemical structure. Beyond that generalization, the following are competing theories:

1) Influence on the actual numbers of intestinal bacteria. Low level consumption of antibiotics can change the species makeup of the bacterial population.

2) Influence metabolism of the bacteria and the host. By killing off bacteria that produce toxins, a healthier environment for beneficial bacteria can be maintained. The antibiotics themselves may be absorbed and affect the metabolism of the host animal.

3) Nutrient sparing effect. Glucose and carbohydrates are spared, thus more are available for absorption by the animal. Increased or decreased absorption of amino acids, minerals and vitamins that are available for absorption by the animal. And increased or decreased organic acid production occur.

4) Influence the thickness of the intestinal wall. Bacteria can irritate the intestinal walls by producing toxins. This irritation results in thicker walls. By preventing the production of toxins, there is less irritation and nutrients are more efficiently absorbed by thinner, healthier walls.

5) Disease prevention. Mild or subclinical infections are treated and cured, improving overall health.

Recently, controversy has arisen because of the increase of human pathogens (harmful organisms) that are antibiotic resistant. It is likely that increasing pressure from an alarmed public and medical community will result in antibiotics no longer being used as growth promotants.

EXAMPLES OF GROWTH-INDUCING ANTIBIOTICS

The following are used for growth promotion in the food industry:
Bacitracin, Bambermycins, Chloretetracycline, Erythromycin, Monensin, Lincomycin, Oxtetracycline, Penicillin, Tylosin, Virginiamycin, Flavomycin and Spiramycin.[2]

BODYBUILDING APPLICATIONS

For bodybuilders, a daily dosage in the milligram range, as part of a heavy training schedule, might produce the AGE. If you are also taking anabolic steroids, the antibiotics may possibly impede their effect. In the liver, many of these drugs are deactivated via conjugation (the steroid molecule is linked to a sugar molecule called glucuronic acid). Some of these steroid glucuronides enter the bile and flow into the small intestine. The normal bacterial flora (population and type) of the gut will hydrolyze (via microbial glucuronidase) the new compounds back to the parent steroid. The drug can then be reabsorbed and repeat its action.[3]

The downside to all this is that antibiotics can kill off many of the beneficial bacteria. Or worse you could create a whole strain of antibiotic-resistant bacteria. The question you have to ask is: "Is it worth it just for a few more pounds of muscle mass?" We strongly suggest leaving antibiotics to physicians and the food industry.

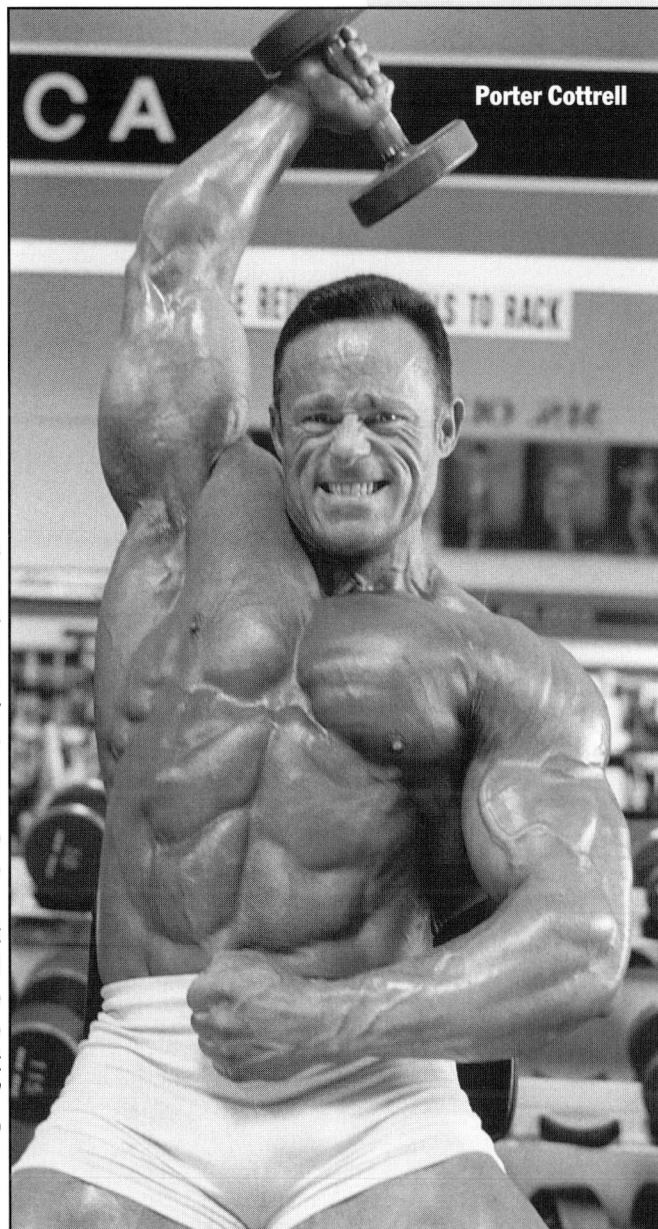

Porter Cottrell

References
1) Grant, R. An Overview On Growth Promotants, in Powers, J. and Powers, T. *The Use of Drugs in Food Animal Medicine*, Proceedings of the Tenth Annual Food Animal Conference, Ohio State Univeristy Press, Columbus, 1984.
2) Hoffmann, B. Introductory Remarks To Beta-Agonists And Their Effects On Growth And Carcass Quality in Farm Animals, in Hanrahan, J., ed. Beta-Agonists and Their Effects on Animal Growth and Carcass Quality, A Seminar in the CEC Program of Coordination and Research in Animal Husbandry, held in Brussels,19 to 20, May 1987, Elsevier Applied Science Publishers Ltd., Essex, 1987.
3) Arnold, P. Ask Patrick Arnold, Mesomorphosis Interactive, http://www.mesomorphosis.com/departments/arnold/current.htm, July, 1998.

CHAPTER SIX

Ecdysteroids: The Latest Anabolics?

Ecdysteroids are substances found in insects and crustaceans that are primarily involved in the molting process.[1, 2] In insects, a brain hormone activates the prothoracic glands, to produce the growth and differentiation (molting) hormone. The active part of this hormone is a ketone containing 18-carbon molecule called ecdysone. This hormone has more than one form. Ecdysones stimulate the molting process and immediately initiate an increase in epidermal (outer skin layer) protein, ribonucleic acid (RNA), mitochondria and endoplasmic reticulum (ER).[7] In plants, ecdysteroids (called phytoecdysteroids) are found in concentrations that are several orders of magnitude higher than in insects.[2] The role of phytoecdysteroids in plant physiology is not fully understood, but it is theorized that their presence was an evolutionary adaptation to protect the plant from insect predators. Of particular interest to bodybuilders is the anabolic effect that phytoecdysteroids have in vertebrates.[1]

Some plants, long known for their healing effects, were later found to have a rich source of ecdysteroids. One of these is the Asiatic medicinal plant Leuzea (Rhaponticum) carthamoides, also called Iljin (root of the deer Maralu), whose anabolic properties (among others) were known long before it was discovered that this plant was one of the richest sources of ecdysteroids. In 1974, a drug prepared from Luezea was tested on a number of domestic animals. The effects reported were: stimulation of metabolism, enhanced muscular functions, increased body growth, improved nerve activity and pronounced anabolic effects. Three years later, the compound responsible for most of the effects (including anabolic) was identified as 20E (abbreviation for 20-hydroxyecdysone, also called ecdysterone).[1]

Even though ecdysteroids are considered hormones in insects and crustaceans, these chemicals may occupy other another role in the vertebrates. This is because ecdysteroids stimulate already existing biological processes. But they don't appear to be able to act as rate limiting factors of growth, nor are they synthesized in the body. Therefore, they cannot be considered to be hormones in vertebrates.

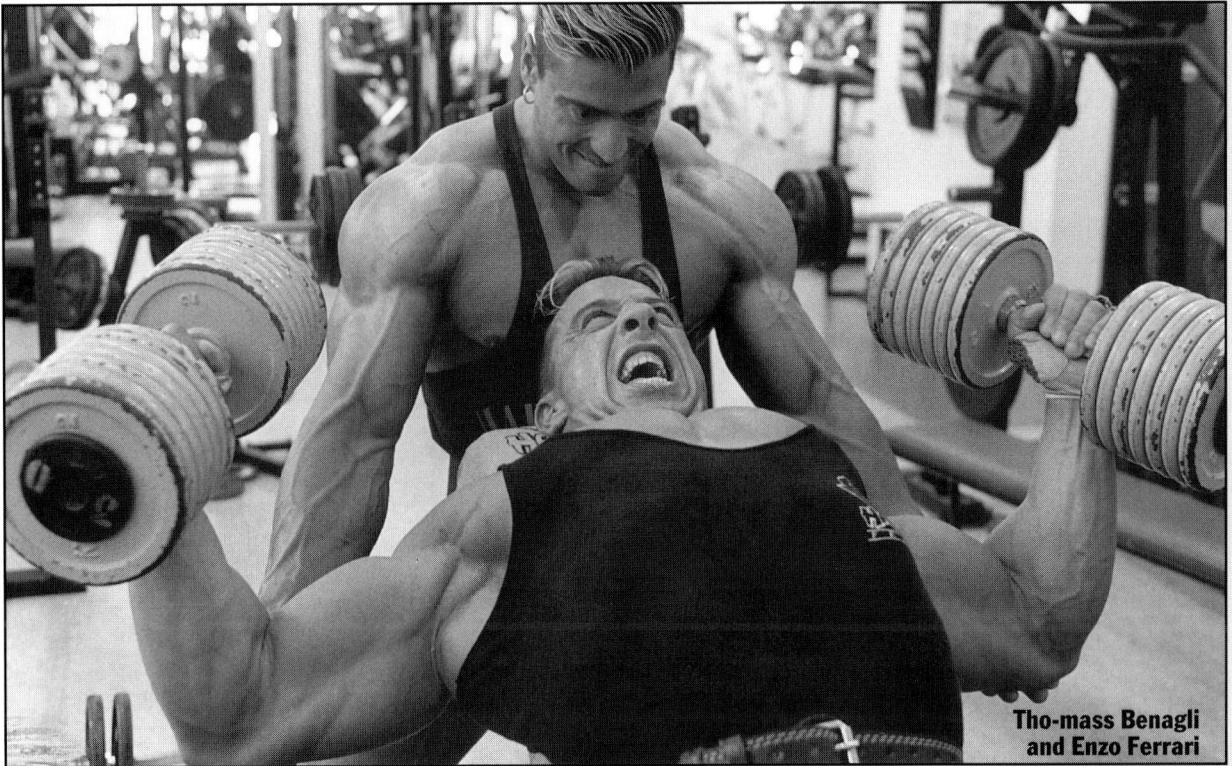

Tho-mass Benagli and Enzo Ferrari

So what are they? The answer appears to be in both their structural make up and role. In insects the molecular arrangement is very specific, and involved primarily in the molting process. In plants and animals the molecule is more general in nature, and the substance plays a role in a number of different physiological responses. For example, besides the previously discussed anabolic actions, ecdysteroids have antitumor properties. So while there is disagreement among biochemists as to their exact classification, the general consensus is that grouping ecdysteroids with essential vitamins might be a good idea.[1]

THE RUSSIAN CONNECTION

One of the most interesting observations about ecdysteroids is that animals grow more, while eating less food of lower quality. This spurred agriculture officials in the former Soviet Union to use Leuzea as an ideal food additive for livestock. Indeed, large experiments were carried out in which the pulverized green parts of Leuzea were fed to cattle, with pronounced anabolic effects. Further studies with mice, rats, pigs and quail have all reported similar results. The quail study was of particular interest, because it compared subjects that received pure 20E without Leuzea in the diet, with subjects that consumed Leuzea seeds of the same 20E content. The results were almost identical, thus proving three things:

1) That 20E was the ecdysteroid responsible for the anabolic effects.[1]
2) Leuzea seeds could be used as an effective and cheap supplement, as opposed to pure 20E, which can be horrendously expensive. The other good news is that one kilogram of Leuzea seed can contain 20 grams of 20E. The plant is non-toxic and ecdysteroids themselves have no harmful effects on mammals. In other words, Luezea seeds are safe to eat.

3) Bodybuilders with digestive problems who limit their caloric intake, those who cannot afford high-quality supplements and anyone dieting down for a competition, may still be able to experience anabolic effects even while reducing their food intake.

The National Research Institute of Sport in Moscow, Russia (the primary organization for sports research and development for the Russian Olympic teams) carried out a study on the synergistic effects of a protein supplement containing Leuzea carthamoides extracts. The combination was optimal in achieving the highest increase in work capacity among athletes. Also recorded were an increase in muscle and a significant decrease in bodyfat. Despite the strong anabolic effects observed, the extract produced no side effects in any of the subjects.

Claude Groulx

Numerous Russian laboratory studies have repeatedly shown the anabolic properties of Leuzea carthamoides. These include: the capacity to increase bodyweight by improving the muscle to fat ratio, increasing both hemoglobin and erythrocyte levels, increasing protein content in the blood and a reduction of uric acid. The proven net result is that the body's anabolic processes outpace the catabolic processes; leading to greater fitness, endurance and performance.[8]

There are also commercial preparations available. Ecdisten was obtained from the roots of Leuzea carthamoides. Developed by the Institute of Natural Compounds, at the Uzbek Academy of Sciences in Tashkent, it was the first ecdysteroid-based drug, marketed by Medexport, in Moscow. Available since 1982, it is sold in pill form – each pill containing five milligrams of 20E equivalent. Independent analysis confirmed 4.3 milligrams, of which 20E is the major constituent. The recommended dosage is one or two pills orally, three times a day, for 15 to 20 days. Break for one to two weeks and repeat the cycle (if you wish).[1]

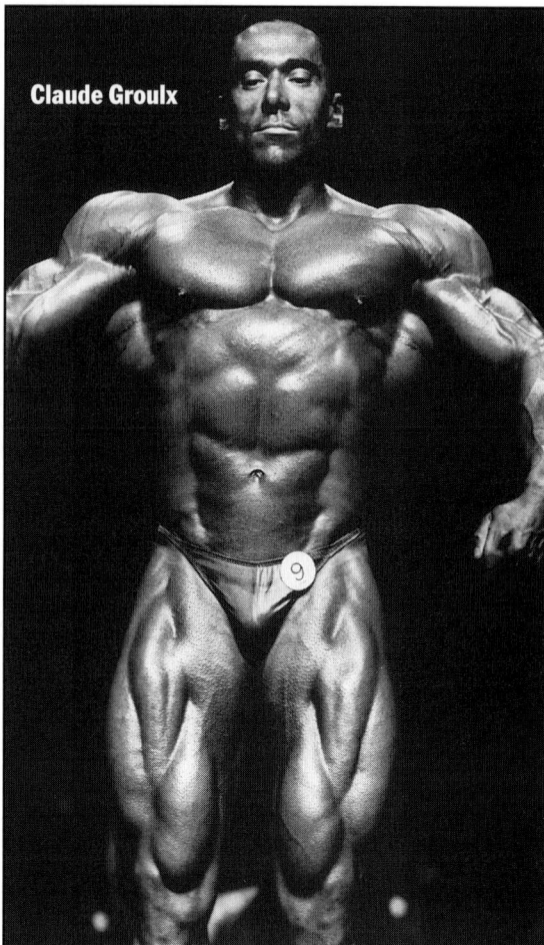

ANABOLIC TEA

Maralan is a Czech tea made from the green parts of Leuzea carthamoides (0.8 to 0.22 percent 20E content), and sold in the Czech Republic. Leuzea drops an alcohol-based root extract, with high concentrations of ecdysteroids. It is sold in both the Czech and Slovak Republics. Both products are advertised as having rejuvenating effects, and based on the previous information, we would expect they would have anabolic effects as well.[1]

ONE WORD OF CAUTION

A complicating issue in using herbal preparations is the nature of the ecdysteroids themselves. They exist in a dynamic state within the plant. Concentration levels can change with the time of day, physiological stage, age and season. Thus the time of harvest is crucial in maximizing the benefits of a high concentration of 20E. For example, to obtain maximal levels of 20E in the whole plant when harvesting Leuzea carthamoides, one must harvest:

1) At 7:00 a.m. or 11:00 p.m.
2) During the rapid growth phase.
3) In the autumn.[2]

It might get you more bang for your buck by buying Leuzea carthamoides seeds. Using the Ecdisten dosage, we suggest the following cycle:

Take one-fourth to half a gram of Leuzea seeds, three times a day for 15 to 20 days. You will actually get more 20E than if you were taking Ecdisten. Since this is a very tiny amount, and the seeds are non-toxic, you can easily afford to increase the dosage if you wish. To assist the digestive process, you might want to put them through a coffee grinder before you eat them. This will give the stomach acids more surface area to work on.

How cheap is this form of 20E compared to pure pharmaceutical preparations?

SOURCE	AMOUNT OF 20E	COST (US DOLLARS)
Leuzea seeds	1 kg (20 to 30 g of 20E)[1]	
Companies:		
Aldrich	10 mg	$90.95
Sigma	10 mg	$90.95
Fluka	10 mg	$231.00
ICN	10 mg	$ 200.70
Biotechnologia Sblk	5 mg	$25.50
Latroxan	10 mg	$59.00
Northern Biochemical	25 mg	$195.30
Scitech	10 mg	$55.00[3]

References
1) Slama, K. and Lafont, R. Insect hormones – ecdysteroids: Their presence and actions in vertebrates, *European Journal of Entomology*, 92, 355-377, 1995.
2) Lafont, R., Bouthier, A., and Wilson, I. Phytoecdysteroids: Structures, Occurrence, Biosynthesis and Possible Ecological Significance, *Proc. Conf. Insect Chem. Ecol., Tabor*, 1990, 197-214, Academia Prague and SPB Acad. Publ., The Hague, 1991.
3) Lafont, R. Commercial sources for ecdysteroids, *Announcement*, Ecole Normale Superieure, Department de Biologie, CNRS URA 686, 46 rue díUlm, 75230 Paris cedex 05, France, Dec.15, 1994.
4) Slama, K., Koudela, K., Tenora, J. and Mathova, A. Insect hormones in vertebrates: Aanabolic effects of 20-hydroxyecdysone in Japanese quail, *Experientia 52*, Birkhauser Verlag, CH-4010 Basel/Switzerland, 1996.
5) Detmar, M., Dumas, M., Bonte, F., Meybeck, A. and Orfanos, C. Effects of ecdysterone on the differentiation of normal human keratinocytes in vitro, Investigative Report, European Journal of Dermatology, 4: 558-62, 1994.
6) *Russian Translation*
7) Patton, R.: *Intoductory Insect Physiology*, W.B. Saunders Company, Philadelphia, 1963.
8) Prime Quest Products: *What Are Adaptogens?*, http://www.stressedout.com/Stressed.html.

CHAPTER SEVEN

Testosterone Precursors and Related Compounds

"Simply that we have a lot more questions than answers regarding such compounds, yet certain companies are selling them without letting people know about these questions. They act as if we know everything there is to know about them as it relates to their effects on people taking them. This lack of honesty bothers me."

– Will Brink, regular *MuscleMag International* columnist, offering his opinion on testosterone precursors and related compounds.

It's safe to say the dominating topic in supplement news over the last half of 1998 was androstenedione and other testosterone boosters. It started in probably the most unlikely of sports – baseball. The year of Mark McGuire was 1998. The St. Louis slugger trashed one of baseball's greatest records – 61 home runs hit by Roger Maris in 1961. And McGuire didn't just hit 62. He finished the year with 70, including two on the last day of the season.

One of the supplements Mark used was androstenedione. Andro is banned in football (ironic given that football has one of the highest rates of steroid use of any sport) and in the Olympics, but as of yet it remains legal in baseball. Andro belongs to a group of substances known as testosterone precursors. And right now they're the hottest topic in athletics.

WHAT THEY ARE

Testosterone precursor is a catchall term to describe any substance that can be converted by the body into the anabolic hormone testosterone. Biochemists use the term intermediates to describe such substances. And although other precursors don't convert to testosterone, but instead into nandrolone – a close cousin of the male hormone – we will also discuss them in this chapter.

With the crackdown on anabolic steroids, supplement manufacturers began looking for substances to take the place of the now illegal drugs. One area of research focused on using natural compounds that the body could convert into testosterone. Other substances allegedly prolong the action of existing testosterone. Unfortunately, many of the substances hyped and promoted as testosterone boosters have little or no scientific backing behind them. So while the anecdotal evidence looks promising, forget trying to track down medical studies that actually scrutinize such substances.

In the following chapter we'll look at the various substances making headlines in bodybuilding gyms and magazines these days. We will do our best not to promote one or the other, but simply give you the scoop on each one and let you make up your own mind.

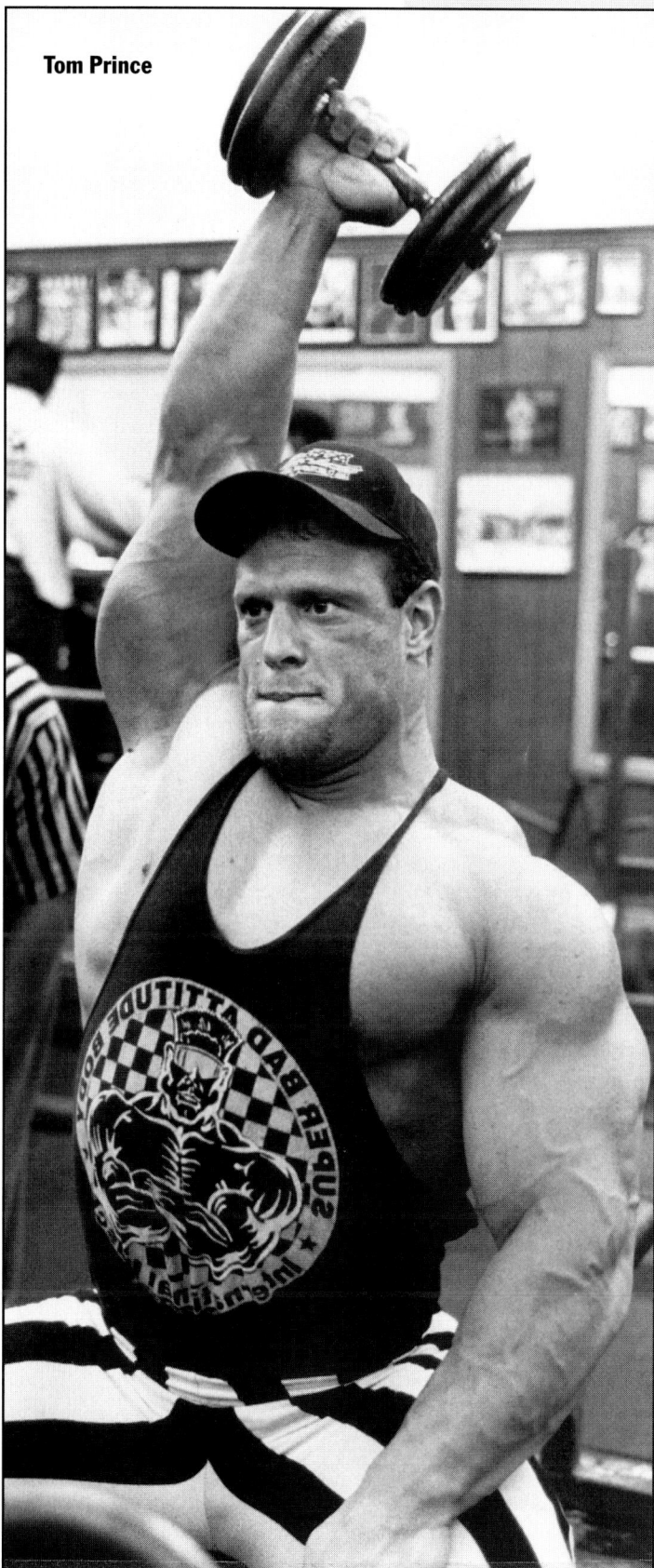

BIOCHEM 101

Before diving into the actual supplements, we need to briefly discuss some general biochemistry. We promise to be gentle, but a couple of points will touch on organic chemistry. This is necessary given the molecular arrangement of many of the substances we will be looking at. When Robert Kennedy said in the *Anabolic Primer* that MuscleMag International might soon need a biochemist on staff, he wasn't kidding. The biochemistry tossed around by supplement manufacturers these days would frighten most bodybuilders from the 1950s and 1960s.

TESTOSTERONE PRECURSOR CLASSIFICATION

Testosterone precursors can be generally divided into two categories – "4" and "5" steroid molecules. Now the organic chemists out there are starting to cringe, but for our purposes this is detailed enough. The designation 4 and 5 refers to the position of a chemical double bond. Basically atoms like to have a full compliment of electrons. When an atom has a lone electron, it shares electrons with another similar atom. Chemists represent such sharing on paper with two parallel lines (indicating a bond) connecting the two atoms. Atoms with the full compliment of electrons also share, but the bond is represented by a single straight line.

Besides the absence or presence of a double bond, biochemists like to indicate where the double bond is located. Test precursors with the double bond in the fourth position on the molecule chain are called "4," and those with the double bond in the fifth position are called "5."

The following is from a 1998 issue of the online drug/supplement magazine *Testosterone.*[14] It divides some of the common precursors into the two categories.

Tom Prince

PRECURSOR STEROIDS IN THE 4 CATEGORY

Testosterone
Progesterone
Androstenedione
4-androstenediol
19-nortestosterone

PRECURSOR STEROIDS IN THE 5 CATEGORY

DHEA
Pregnenolone
5-androstenediol
19-nor 5-androstenediol

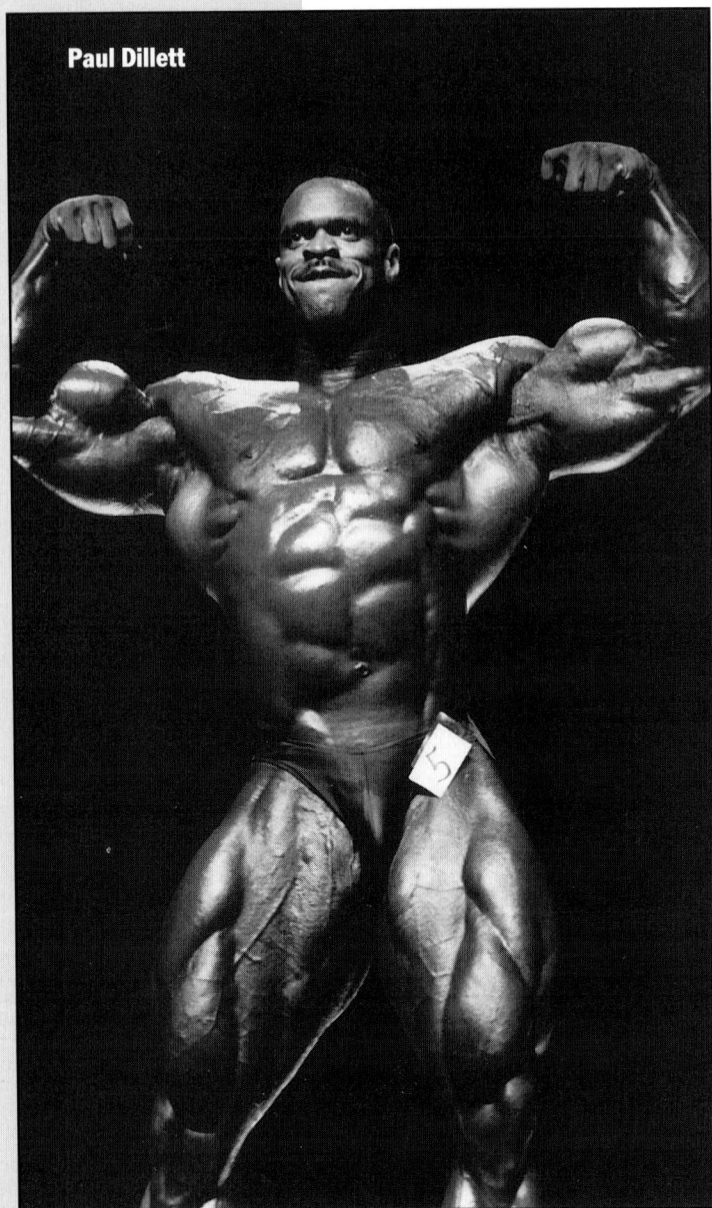

Paul Dillett

WHAT'S THE BIG DEAL?

According to some researchers 4 precursors are more effective than 5s because the 5s must be converted to 4s before being converted to testosterone. In short, that double bond we were making such a big deal over must be switched from the fifth to the fourth position, before testosterone can be produced.

Of course there's much more involved than a simple bond switching. And as mentioned earlier, some of the precursors don't even convert to testosterone, but to nandrolone (the active ingredient in the anabolic steroid deca-durabolin). Finally, some work by naturally boosting testosterone production or slowing its breakdown. When evaluating the following substances, please be aware that you're reading about a topic that is evolving at an alarming rate. What's accepted today maybe outdated next month.

ANDROSTENEDIONE

It's only appropriate to start this chapter with the one substance that has brought testosterone precursors to the forefront. When word first broke that baseball great Mark McGuire was using andro, supplement stores couldn't keep the product on their shelves. This is ironic as, in bodybuilding circles, andro was on its way out.

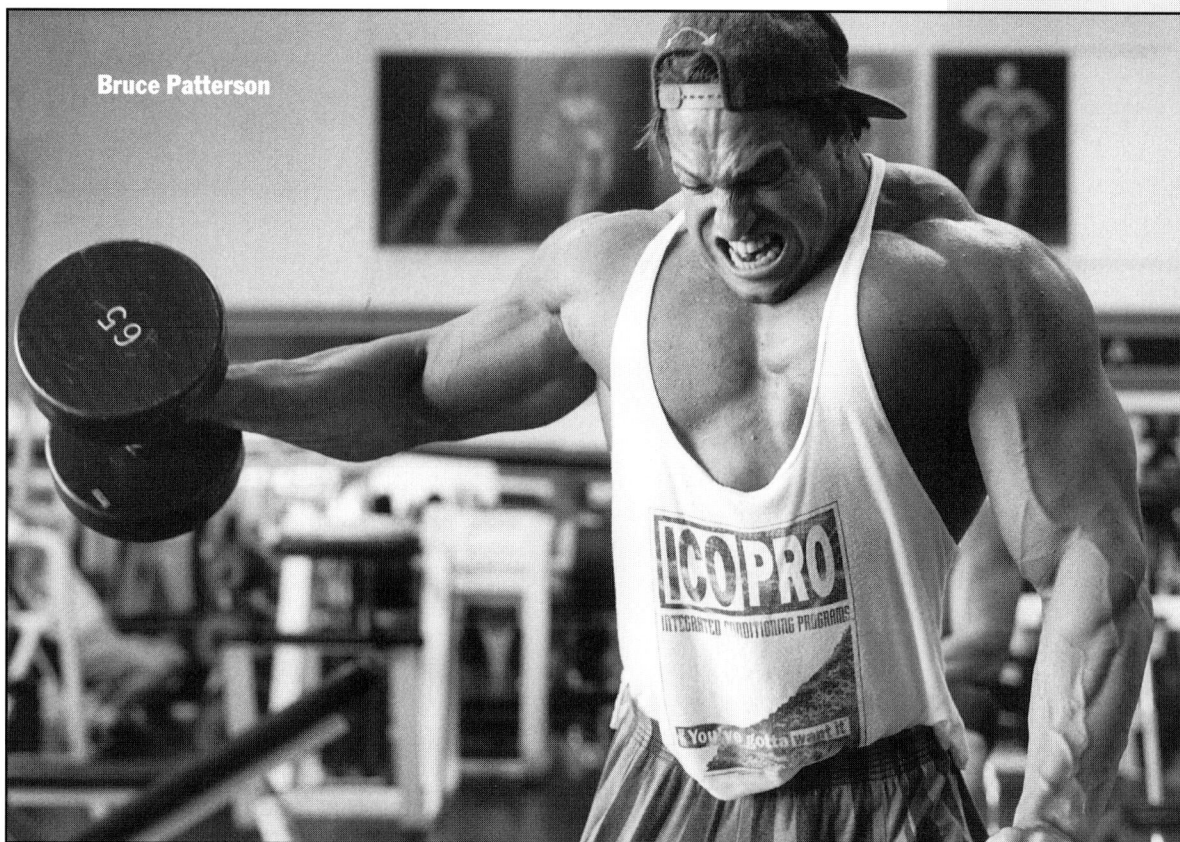

Bruce Patterson

A LEFTOVER FROM THE IRON CURTAIN

Andro got its first big break from research carried out in the former East Germany. With success in athletics being part of the communist statement, athletic researchers were always on the lookout for substances that could boost performance, but not be detected in a drug test. According to declassified reports from the East German doping program, many of the athletes were using an andro nasal spray that would boost testosterone levels for only a few hours – enough to increase performance, but not enough to fail a drug test. We'll never know just how effective such supplements were, but the science of testosterone precursors had begun.

Androstenedione is an intermediate precursor to testosterone. In theory this sounds great, but there's a host of variables that must occur for andro to be converted into the desired hormone. Even when all the necessary variables are present, andro is not all it's cracked up to be. Most marketers say it increases testosterone levels, and leave it at that. What they don't tell you is only a small amount (10 to 20 percent is the range most commonly quoted) is converted from andro to testosterone. Also, andro only stays active in the system for a short period of time, say a few hours. Biochemically speaking, andro has a short half-life (the time needed for half the substance to degrade or be converted into another substance). We also must point out that there's little research to suggest slightly elevated testosterone levels can make a significant impact on athletic performance. A few capsules a day is probably not going to lead to any meaningful muscle growth. Unless you were to continuously consume andro every couple of hours, you are unlikely to see any major effects.

Keep in mind, that testosterone is only one of the end products of andro metabolism. Andro can also be converted into estrogen. Even though there's limited evidence that estrogen can stimulate testosterone levels, there's more evidence to show that higher estrogen levels lead to increased fat storage (one of the primary reasons why women on average have higher fat levels than men).

Lee Apperson

SIDE EFFECTS

Andro is in a different category than many harsher anabolic steroids; especially when it comes to producing unwanted side effects. Still, there are risks. In many users andro can increase facial and torso acne. Remember testosterone and its derivatives also have androgenic effects (development of the secondary sex characteristics, hair growth, etc). The reason acne is common in the teenage years, especially males, is because of high levels of testosterone. If you had severe or even moderate acne as a teenager then taking andro puts you at risk.

If there's one side effect that may offer an athletic edge it's elevated aggression levels. It's common knowledge that elevated testosterone levels are related to aggression. Numerous studies with prisoners have confirmed this (of course there are many more variables that lead to incarceration). For athletes in a sport requiring mental aggressiveness, andro may offer a slight edge.

A less common, but potentially more severe, side effect concerns andro's effects on the prostate gland. This small organ, located in the lower groin region of males, is very susceptible to high androgen levels. In fact, many men (20 to 25 percent) will naturally have prostate problems later in life. Taking any substance that's biochemically similar (or in the case of andro, possibly converted) to testosterone, increases the risk of prostate problems, including cancer.

Finally, assuming andro actually does get converted to testosterone, you have to deal with feedback interference. Most of the body's hormones, including testosterone, are regulated by a biofeedback mechanism. In effect, the body increases or decreases levels depending on how much of the hormone is circulating. As soon as you add an outside source, the body's natural hormonal axis is disrupted.

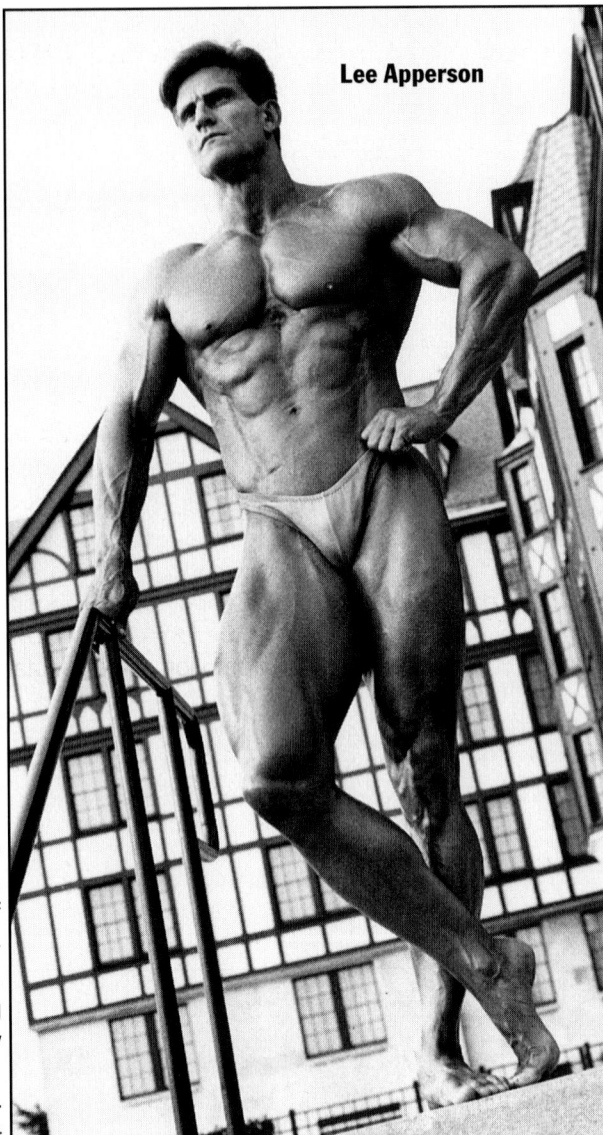

HOW MUCH?

With little scientific evidence available, dosage recommendation is basically a shot in the dark. The accepted dosage is 100 to 200 milligrams per day – preferably spread over three or four smaller dosages. This is probably enough to slightly elevate testosterone levels (but as we said earlier, how relevant this is we don't know) without producing the unwanted side effects. The bottom line, however, depends on the individual. If you have a history of hair loss, prostate problems or acne in your family, then we strongly advise against using andro products.

DEHYDROEPIANDROSTERONE – DHEA

DHEA is another substance found on the road to testosterone production. Although not as close to testosterone as andro, evidence suggests that more DHEA is converted to the active hormone, testosterone than with andro.

DHEA is secreted by the cortex of the adrenal glands (two small structures located on top of the kidneys). As with most hormones, DHEA is secreted in response to another hormone secreted by the brain, in this case adrenocorticotropic hormone (ACTH). DHEA and testosterone are similar in that the body starts secreting them early in life. They peak in the late teens and early 20s, and then decline with age. Because of this relationship, there's much research ongoing to determine if DHEA can be used to combat some of the deterioration that takes place with age. Since DHEA can be converted into testosterone, supplement manufacturers are going all out in their promotion of the substance as an athletic supplement.

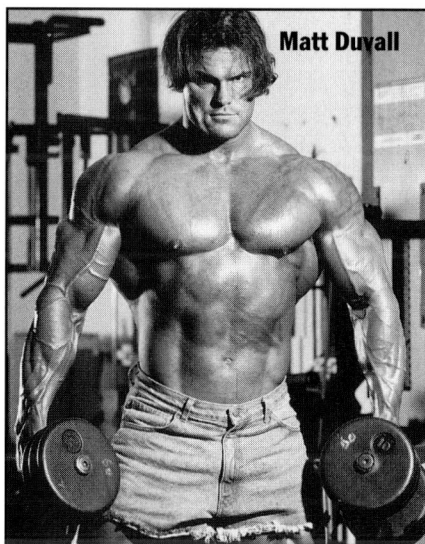

THE LATEST RESEARCH

Matt Duvall

It has been known for some time now that animals fed a calorie restricted diet, live longer than animals fed a normal diet. Research has also determined that DHEA levels decline with age (by some estimates down to 10 percent by age 70). One recent study published in the *Journal of Clinical Endocrinology and Metabolism* looked at the relationship between calorie restriction, aging and DHEA levels. A group of 74 monkeys were fed a calorie-reduced diet and then examined for DHEA levels. While the control group (non-restricted group) showed the expected DHEA decline, the restricted group had levels higher than expected. The researchers concluded that decreasing DHEA levels is one of the variables responsible for the symptoms of aging.[1]

Given the previous, it's not surprising that researchers are looking for ways to naturally boost DHEA levels, or to slow down its decline with aging. A recent study published in the *Journal of Nutritional Biochemistry* offers one suggestion. Researchers looked at the relationship between vitamin E, the mineral selenium and DHEA. As theorized, rats fed a diet deficient in vitamin E and selenium had reduced DHEA levels in the adrenal

"Just to make sure I wasn't missing all the incredible research on this muscle supplement, I called every supplier I could get numbers for and asked them for their scientific support. Got a lot of uhs, but no research. Not even a pliable rational. It's all speculation."

– Dr. Bob Lefavi, in an article for *All Natural Muscular Development Magazine*, commenting on the unknown element with nor-19 and diol-6.

"Since this product has just come off the grey market, no official human studies have been conducted on 19-nor. However, I have talked with numerous competitive bodybuilders and powerlifters who have been using it. The number one result I hear is that athletes are getting stronger and larger with each workout."

– Ken Wells, *MuscleMag International* contributor, commenting on the latest ergogenic aid for bodybuilders, nor-19.

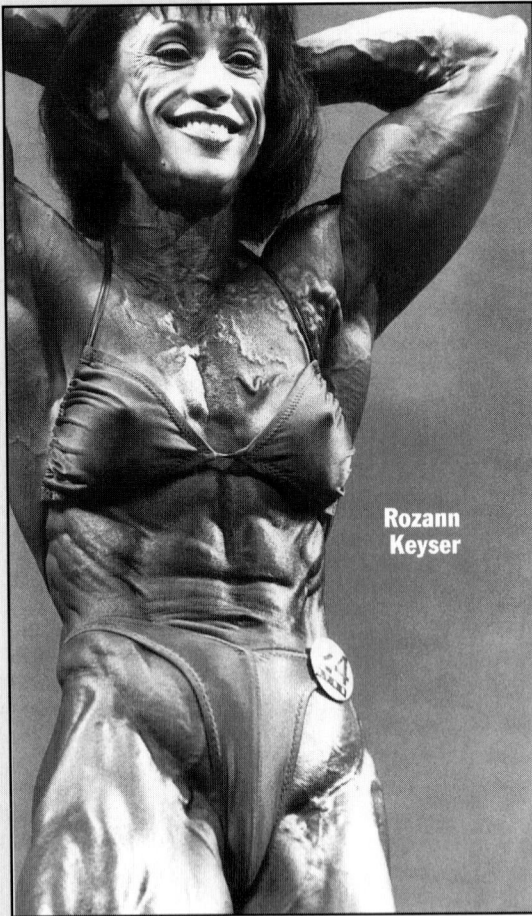

Rozann
Keyser

cortex. Surprisingly only rats with restricted Vitamin E levels had reduced DHEA levels in the brain. Selenium deficiency didn't appear to effect brain DHEA levels. Now to the crucial part of the experiment. When the same rats were fed normal amounts of vitamin E and selenium, their adrenal DHEA levels returned to normal.[2]

DHEA research has also found that it's not just athletes who may benefit from DHEA supplementation. Recent studies with post-menopausal women who took DHEA for three months had increased levels of insulin-like growth factor 1 (IGF-1). The researchers concluded that DHEA could reverse some of the problems experienced by older women due to declining estrogen levels.[3]

Another study published in the *Journal of Nutritional Biochemistry* looked at the role DHEA plays in the immune system. Older mice given DHEA supplements and antioxidants had T-Cell counts significantly higher than non-supplemented mice.[4] Further, mice infected with viruses had a greater immune response when they received DHEA supplementation.

T-Cells are one of the immune system's primary soldiers in the fight against invading pathogens (viruses, bacteria, parasites, etc). As people age, their T-Cell levels fall, leaving them susceptible to any parasite that comes along. Diseases that would be non-life threatening earlier in life now become deadly. Just think of the number of elderly individuals who die each year from pneumonia. Most healthy individuals never get this common ailment, and those that do usually kick it out of their systems in a week or so. But to an elderly person with a weakened immune system, such bacteria can be deadly. The previous study offers hope that a simple supplement may keep the immune system up to youthful fighting trim.

HOW MUCH?

As with androstenedione, nailing down a precise DHEA dosage for athletes is tricky at best. If you go by the gym scuttlebutt, males should take 100 to 200 milligrams per day, while women can get by on as little as 25 milligrams per day. *MuscleMedia* publisher Bill Phillips states that he's talked to bodybuilders who have megadosed on the stuff (more than 1000 milligrams per day), but seen little added benefit. It seems a couple 100 milligrams a day will either do it or not. Taking more makes little sense. For women readers, keep in mind DHEA could boost your testosterone levels considerably. In fact on a proportion basis, women will probably get more out of DHEA than men. This is great from the athletic side of things, but don't forget the androgenic effects we mentioned earlier. Extra body hair and deeper voices are not things most women desire.

As a final comment, those athletes involved in drug tested events should be aware that DHEA can alter the six to one testosterone to epitestosterone ratio used by the IOC (International Olympic Committee) and other athletic federations. Even though this ratio test is loaded with faults, failure means an automatic positive test for anabolic steroids.

NORANDROTESTENEDIONEL (NOR-19) AND NORANDROSTENEDIOL

NOTE – Most of the following information was obtained from MuscleTech, the most prominent supplement manufacturer endorsing Nor-19 and Diol-5. Both supplements have a very poor record in scientific journals. This is not to say they've been proven useless. But as popular supplements go, Nor-19 and Diol-5 don't have the immaculate scientific pedigree of glutamine or creatine (both of which have been proven to improve athletic performance). The next year will either see both supplements fade into history like dibencocide (for our younger readers check out some muscle magazines from the mid-80s), or become the foundation for the next generation of bodybuilding supplements. Only time will tell.

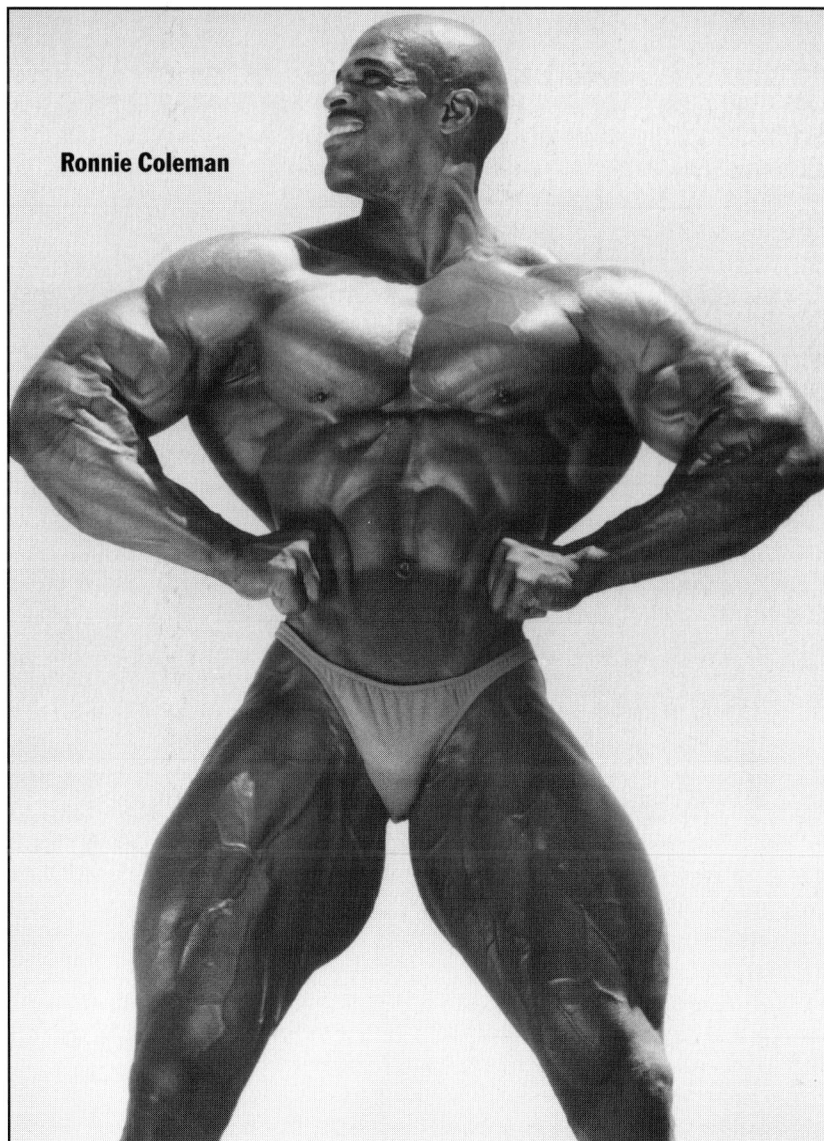

Ronnie Coleman

"For example, more than 70 percent of the 250 NFL players we tested were found to be deficient in both zinc and magnesium."

– Victor Conte of Balco Labs, commenting on a study conducted on NFL football players.

NOR-19 – DECA IN A BOTTLE?

The theory behind Nor-19 is that the liver converts it into nandrolone, the active ingredient in the popular anabolic steroid deca-durabolin (nandrolone deconate).[18] Muscle Tech claims that the conversion rate is approximately 5.61 percent.

Frank Sepe

The reason that Muscle Tech (and others such as Meritech and Euthenics) have focused on nandrolone is because deca-durabolin has a reputation for being one of the safest and most effective anabolic steroids ever invented. In fact, deca is probably the most popular steroid on the black market. Of course this means it's also the most faked drug out there. Supplement manufacturers know its popularity, and are trying to capitalize by offering a cheaper, natural alternative. In theory they may have a point, but the problem is that they are very skimpy on references. Before we endorse such supplements, a couple of important questions need to be answered. First, does the liver in fact convert nor-19 into nandrolone? Second, if nandrolone is produced, is it in an active form? It's one thing for the body to produce a product and another for that product to be bioactive. Finally, if the answer to the previous two questions is yes, how much is produced. As with androstenedione, the body needs a certain amount of a substance for it to increase muscle size and strength. Until such questions are answered by quality scientific research, we suggest holding a moderate degree of skepticism in using nor-19 based supplements.

5-ANDROSTENEDIOL (DIOL-5)

Diol-5 is a close cousin of nor-19, which is also reported to be converted to nandrolone in the liver. It is sold in many countries as methandriol. According to substance manufacturers, diol-5 produces three main effects in the body. First, it's supposedly anticatabolic; meaning it suppresses cortisol and other stress hormones released during intense training. Cortisol causes protein to be leached from muscle tissue, leading to muscle wasting. The higher the cortisol levels, the lower the ability of the body to recover from exercise.

Another proposed property of diol-5 is its ability to bind to estrogen receptors. The more estrogen receptors blocked, the less effects this feminizing hormone will have. Closely related to this, diol-5 also has the ability to prevent the conversion of testosterone to estrogen (called aromatization).

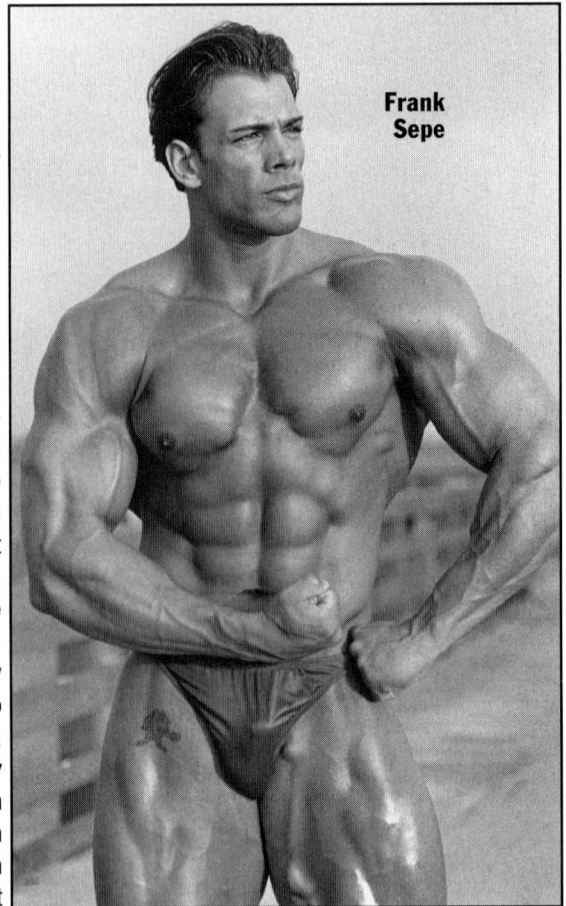

A final benefit of diol-5 is, like glutamine, it can strengthen the immune system by increasing the activation of lymphocytes.[17] As many bodybuilders will admit, a couple months of intense training often leaves them in a drained state and open to every flu or bug that comes along. Diol-5 may boost the immune system, helping to ward off such stress-induced ailments.

HOW MUCH?

Without sounding like a broken record, the dosages worked out for both nor-19 and diol-5 are based on supplement manufacturers and gym talk. The most commonly cited dosages are 100 to 200 milligrams of nor-19, and 50 to 100 milligrams of diol-5 per day. In fact many supplement manufacturers combine the two in one product (i.e. MuscleTech's Nortesten). This supposedly produces a synergistic effect, with both substances boosting the other's effects.

SIDE EFFECTS

If the theory behind nor-19 and diol-5 is sound, and both do in fact get converted to nandrolone, then the incidence of side effects is extremely low. Deca-durabolin is one of the safest anabolic steroids ever produced. Now this flies in the face of what the anti-steroid groups say, but from a medical point of view nandrolone is as safe as it gets (provided it's genuine). It is possible that 20 or 30 years down the road something may show up, but we doubt it. Nor-19 and diol-5 don't produce near the same punch as the steroid equivalent deca. Deca has been around for decades and, as of yet, there's nothing linked to it. We expect the same of nor-19 and diol-5.

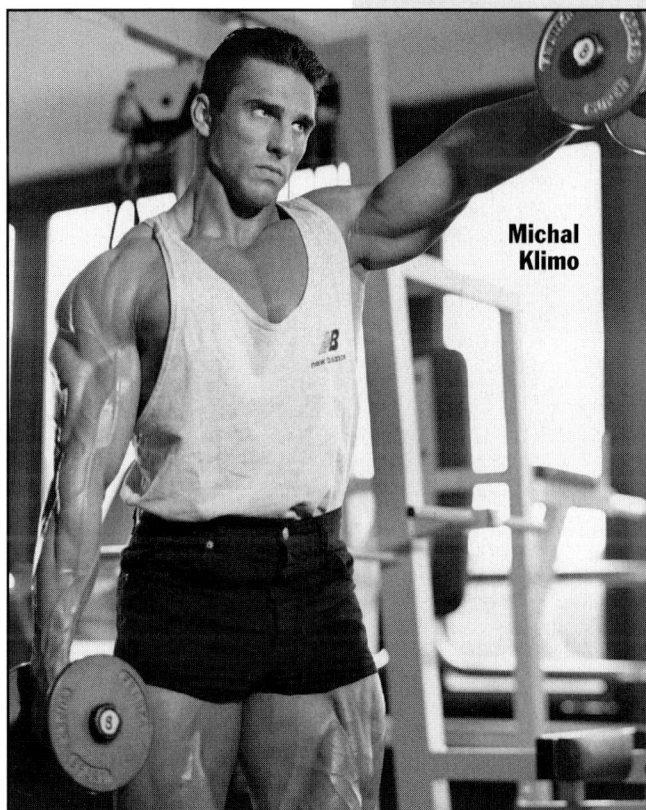

Michal
Klimo

4-ANDROSTENEDIOL – THE BEST OF THE BEST?

4-AD is the brainchild of chemist Patrick Arnold and his company LPJ. 4-AD is promoted as being the best of the current generation of precursors because it converts to testosterone at three times the rate of such other precursors as androstenedione.[15] In one study, presented at a major conference in Finland in late 1998, 100 milligrams of 4-AD was found to raise testosterone 42.5 percent, as compared to only 10.9 percent for an equal amount of androstenedione.[16]

4-AD is found in several tissues of the body including the adrenal cortex, hypothalamus and testes. Besides raising testosterone levels higher than other precursors, 4-AD may have another advantage – it doesn't seem to aromatize to estrogen like many other precursors. Without insulting the biochemists among you, suffice to say 4-AD is missing a side group (in this case a ketone) that most of the others have. Of course the extra testosterone produced by 4-AD can and will aromatize somewhat, but that's the price you pay for playing chemist with your hormone levels.

On paper, 4-AD appears to be the best of the test precursors, but again a degree of skepticism is warranted. The biggest proponents of 4-AD are the same people manufacturing it (although we have to give them credit for using medical references). In fact this is one of the problems with evaluating testosterone precursors. Many of the big bodybuilding magazines have their favorites. Here's a sample:

1) *All Natural Muscular Development* – DHEA
2) *MuscleMag International* (by way of MuscleTech) – Nor-19
3) http://www.testosterone.net ; www.testosterone.net (on-line) – 4-AD
4) *FLEX* – 5-AD

See the problem. No matter how unbiased someone tries to be, it's difficult when there's a financial stake involved. The best piece of advice we can give is to try most of the products and make up your own mind. True this will get pricy. It may set you back many hundreds of dollars to adequately evaluate them all. It then becomes a matter of how much it means to you. If you want to play it safe, stick to the proven supplements like creatine and glutamine until something more concrete comes along pertaining to the precursors.

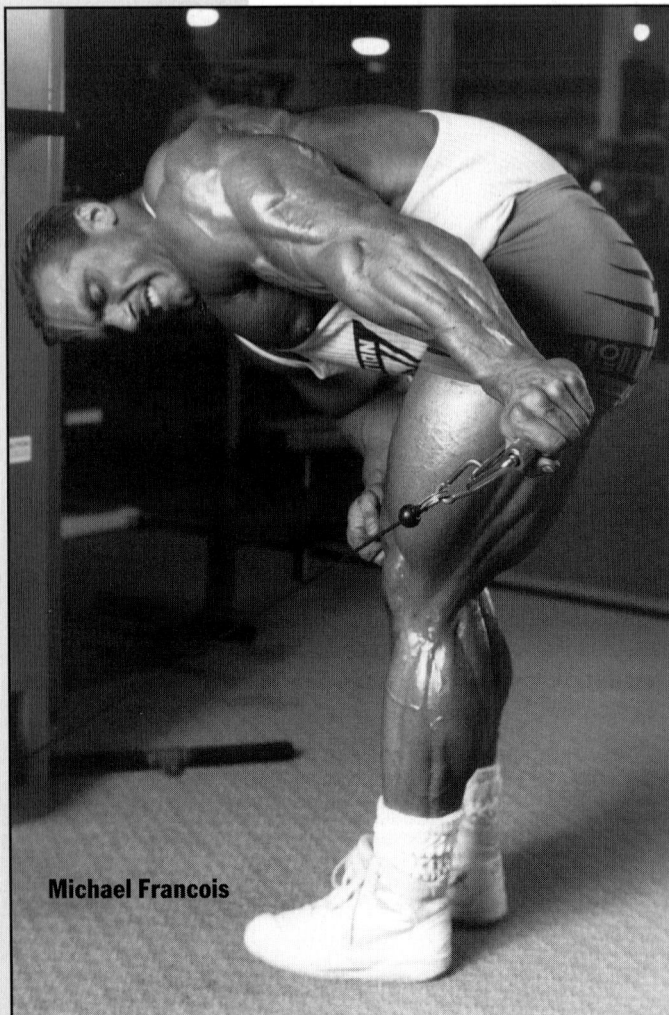
Michael Francois

ZINC

It may surprise many to see zinc included in a chapter on testosterone precursors, but there's a good reason for doing so. Among its many functions, the evidence suggests zinc plays a major role in testosterone production.

Zinc is a mineral that is, despite being needed in trace amounts, involved in virtually hundreds of metabolic actions. Approximately two to three grams of zinc in the body is found within the bones. The rest of the mineral is found mostly in the skin, nails and hair. To give you an idea of zinc's importance, most of the body's hormones such as insulin, estrogen, testosterone and growth hormone, are dependent on zinc. This has been confirmed in recent studies, which suggest hard training athletes may be deficient in zinc.[6] For our female readers you should be aware that birth control pills could also reduce zinc levels. Other evidence linking zinc to testosterone comes from studies with preadolescent males. Researchers found those boys with the highest zinc levels reached puberty faster than those with lower levels.[7]

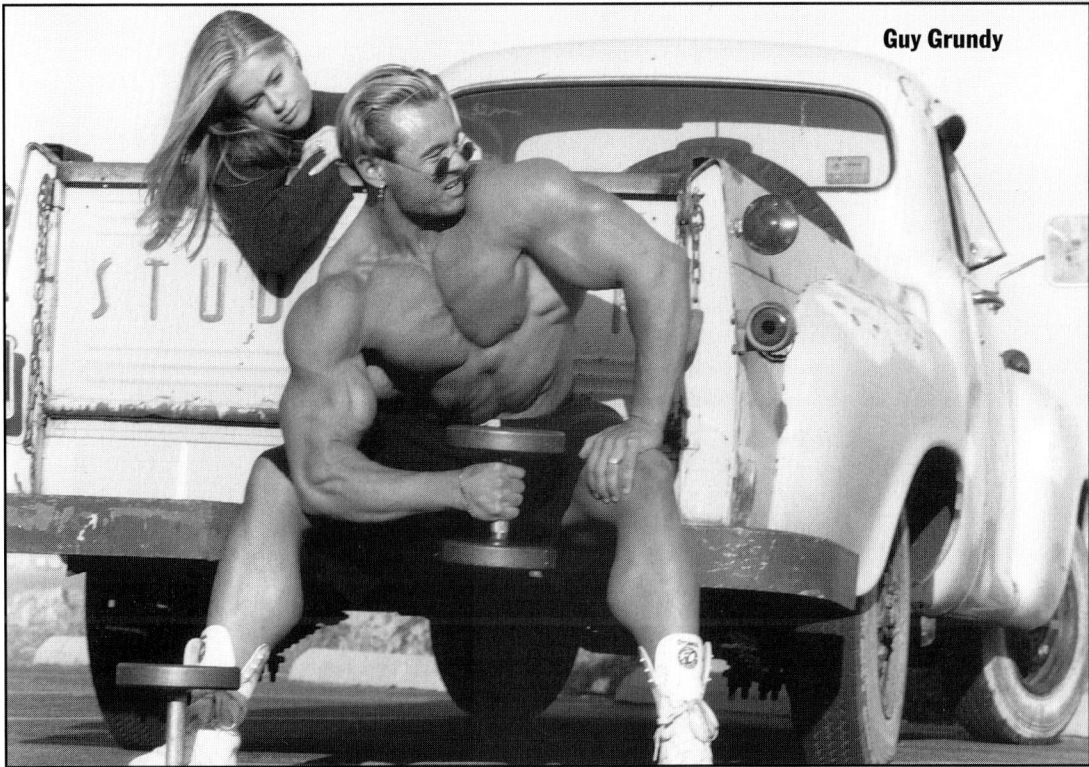

Guy Grundy

We should add that like many common nutrients, zinc will not boost testosterone levels above normal. But if your zinc levels are low (as a hard training athlete you probably fall into this category), then supplementing with zinc insures optimum hormone production.

SIDE EFFECTS

Unless you consume mega doses (500 to 1000 milligrams per day), adverse reactions to zinc are rare. Excessive zinc can interact with other minerals like copper and iron, but this is in extreme cases. Taking 15 to 30 milligrams per day as a supplement is perfectly safe for healthy individuals. In fact, the optimum dosage for hard training athletes is 30 milligrams per day.[13]

CHRYSIN

Chrysin is the common name for a substance obtained from a plant called Passiflora coerulea. Chrysin is an example of a new class of substances called bioflavonoids. Although dismissed for years, recent research suggests bioflavonoids may produce effects in humans. One area of research shows chrysin may offer hope to arthritis sufferers since the substance has anti-inflammatory properties.[8] Other studies show chrysin may have antioxidant properties. Oxidants or free-radicals (no not some free thinkers from the 1960s) are substances that travel through the body, reacting with any molecule with an electrical charge. Such reactions are believed to lead to the degeneration in bodily systems commonly called aging. While not conclusive, chrysin seems to be able to counteract such oxidative damage.[9]

The third area of chrysin research falls into a grey region. Supplement manufacturers promote chrysin as an antiestrogen compound. The substance got its first big boost from supplement/steroid guru Dan Duchaine, who marketed chrysin under the name Flavone X.

The theory behind chrysin is that it prevents the conversion of testosterone to estrogen, thus making more testosterone available.[10] Chrysin is also promoted as being a receptor sensitivity booster. Supposedly chrysin can increase the effectiveness of a given amount of testosterone by making its receptors more sensitive or reactive. The only drawback to the previous is that most of the evidence for it comes from animal studies or invitro (i.e. in a test tube).

HOW MUCH?

With no human studies to go by we can only suggests dosages based on anecdotal evidence. *MuscleMedia* publisher Bill Phillips recommends one to three grams a day, spread over a number of smaller dosages. Comments from bodybuilders who use Chrysin seem to back this up. About all we can say is stick to the previous until some solid science comes along.

TRIBULUS TERRESTRIS

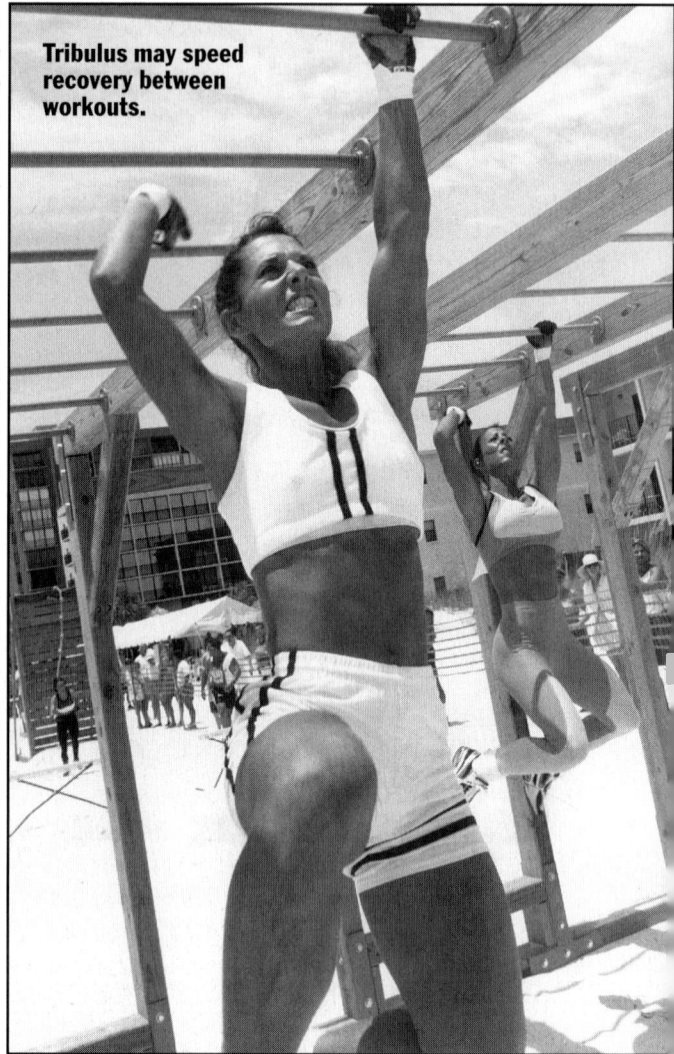

Tribulus may speed recovery between workouts.

Tribulus is one of a growing number of herbs that is getting a lot of press from bodybuilding writers and supplement manufacturers these days. Tribulus has a long history in folk medicine. The ancient Greeks supposedly used is as a diuretic; the Chinese used it to cure just about every ailment known; and Eastern Europeans employ the herb for treating libido.

The reason tribulus has crossed over into bodybuilding is because of the herb's supposed effect on testosterone. Unlike andro and DHEA, which serve as precursors for testosterone, tribulus goes at it from another direction. Tribulus is believed to boost levels of leutinizing hormone (LH). LH is the brain's chemical messenger that tells the testes when to produce more testosterone. So while tribulus doesn't directly increase testosterone levels, it does increase LH levels, which in turn increases testosterone. Now you see why tribulus has been used for thousands of years as an aphrodisiac.

Increasing libido and testosterone is one thing, but many readers are no doubt asking if the herb is of any use to bodybuilders. The answer is a guarded yes. We say guarded because there's limited evidence that tribulus can elevate testosterone levels.[11] One study from England involving strength athletes found that tribulus increased free testosterone levels by an average of 63 percent, and LH levels by 120 percent.[13] Thus, given the relationship between testosterone and muscle building, tribulus may speed recovery between workouts.

USING TRIBULUS

The anecdotal evidence suggests using 500 to 1000 milligrams of tribulus per day. The herb can be taken by itself or, as is the norm these days, combined with a testosterone precursor (andro and DHEA being the most popular).

The only reported side effect from using tribulus is a slight to moderate burning sensation in the stomach. This can easily be eliminated by taking the preparation with meals or copious amounts of water. Finally, pregnant or lactating females should not use tribulus products.

SAW PALMETTO

Saw palmetto is the common name for the tropical plant Serenoa repens. Like tribulus, this palm-like herb has been used for years as an alternative form to mainstream medicine. It too has been promoted to cure just about every physical ailment. And while the scientific evidence is sketchy, few herbs have stood the test of time like Saw palmetto.

Saw palmetto receives its biggest endorsement as an anti-DHT compound. DHT or dihydrotestosterone is one of the metabolites of testosterone, and has been linked to prostate enlargement. Saw palmetto is

Tropical plant, Saw palmetto, is an alternative to mainstream medicine.
– Romeo Villarino

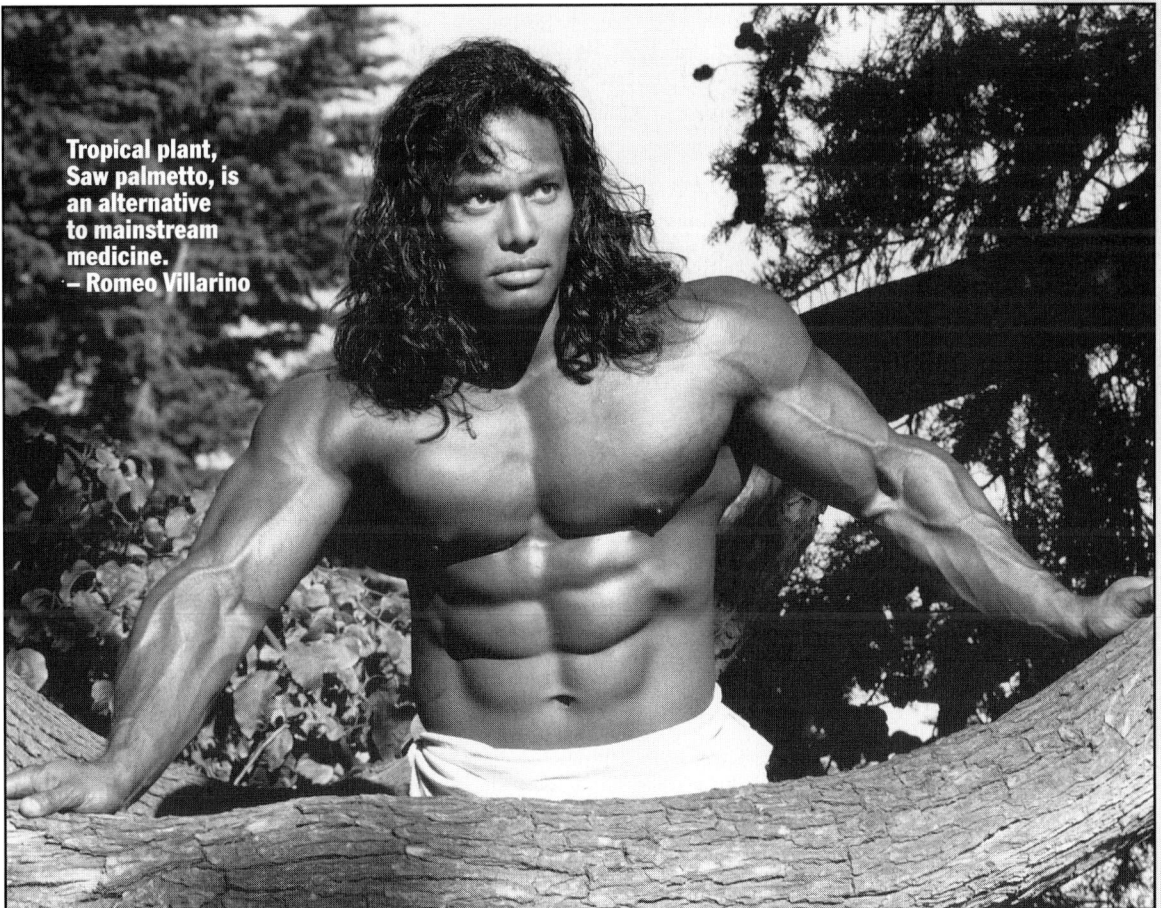

believed to help prevent such conversion. There's also evidence to suggest Saw palmetto extracts are anti-estrogenic in nature.[12] If true, bodybuilders who use steroids or testosterone precursors may want to include Saw palmetto in their supplement arsenal. The recommended dosage is 150 to 200 milligrams per day.

ACETYL-L-CARNITINE (ACL)

This is another substance that received its big break from MuscleTech LTD of Canada. It forms the basis for one of their top selling supplements, Acetabolan.

Acetyl-L-carnitine is the esterfied form of the common fat-transporting substance discussed earlier – carnitine. Approximately 10 percent of carnitine stores are in the acetyl form. While the parent carnitine form helps transport fats in and out of the cell for energy, the esterfied form seems to play a role in raising testosterone levels.

One of the ironic aspects to intense exercise is that when carried to the extreme it can lower testosterone levels – the opposite to what's desired. Stress, of which exercise is one form, has long been known to increase cortisol levels and decrease testosterone levels. Studies with rats have shown that ACL may be able to counteract such catabolism. The exact mechanism of action is not clear, but it is believed ACL increases circulating levels of gonadotropin-releasing hormone. This in turn signals the testes to increase testosterone output.

Now we're not going to say ACL works like steroids (like some advertisers), but the evidence is starting to mount that ACL can play a role in natural ergogenesis. In defense of MuscleTech – the first big supplement manufacturer to promote ACL – most of the rivals that originally criticized ACL have now released their own versions. It seems the early speculation by MuscleTech is starting to be backed up by science.

References
1) Lane, M., Ingram, D., et al. DHEA: A biomarker of primate aging slowed by calorie restriction. *Journal of Clinical Endocrinology and Metabolism*, 82: 7, 2093-2096, 1997.
2) Hu,L., Ng, HP. Dietary selenium and vitamin E affect adrenal and brain DHEA levels in young rats. *Journal of Nutritional Biochemistry*. 9:339-343, 1998.
3) Larkin, M. DHEA: will science confirm the headlines? *The Lancet*, 352: 208, 1998.
4) Jiang,S., Zhang, Z., et al. DHEA synergizes with antioxidant supplements for immune restoration in old as well as retrovirus-infected mice. *The Journal of Nutritional Biochemistry*, 9:362-369, 1998.
5) Lefavi, Bob. The Ultimate All-Natural Testosterone Booster. *All Natural Muscular Development Magazine*, June, 1998.
6) Cordova, A., Alvarez-Mon, M. Behavior of zinc in physical exercise: A special reference to immunity and fatigue. *Neuroscience and Biobehavior Review*, 19:3, 439-445, 1995.
7) Hunt, C.D., et al. Effects of dietary zinc depletion on seminal volume and zinc losss, serum testosterone concentrations, and sperm morphology in young men. *American Journal of Clinical Nutrition*, 56: 148-157, 1992.
8) Tordea, M, et al. Influence of anti-inflammatory flavonoids on degranulation and archidonic acid release in rat neutrophils. *Z. Natruforsch ICI*, 49(3-4) 235-240, 1994.
9) Wolfman, C., et al. Possible anxiolytic effects of chrysin, a central benzodiazepine receptor ligand isolated from passiflora coerulea. *Pharmacologic Biochemical Behavior*, 47 (1) 1-4, 1994.
10) Cambell, D.R., Kurzer, M.S. Flavonoid inhibition of armatase enzyme activity in human preadipocytes, *Journal of Steroid Biochemistry and Molecular Biology*, 46 (3) 381-388, 1993.
11) Wright, J. Sex, a natural wonder, increased sex drive and higher levels of testosterone, All from a herbal preparation, *Muscle and Fitness on Line*, http://www.muscle-fitness.com/sex/tribulus.html.
12) DiSilverio, F., et al. Evidence that Serenoa repens extract displays anti-estrogenic activity in prostatic tissue of benign prostatic hypertrophy. *European Urology*, 21: 309-314, 1992.
13) www.testosterone.net/FEA/html/f10.html.
14) www.testosterone.net/FEA/html/f9.html.
15) Blaquier, J., et al. The amount of testosterone formed upon incubation in human blood. *Endocrinology*, 55, 697-704.
16) Batcheldor, B., and Wright, J. New-age ergogens, *Flex Magazine*, Dec 1998, 227-231.
17) Padgett, D.A., Loria, R.M. In vitro potentiation of lymphocyte activation by dehydroepiandrosterone, androstenediol, and androstenetriol. *Journal of Immunology*, 153 (4) 1544-1552, 1994.
18) Androstenedione et al. Nonprescription Steroids, http://www.physsportsmed.com/issues/1998/11nov/news.htm.

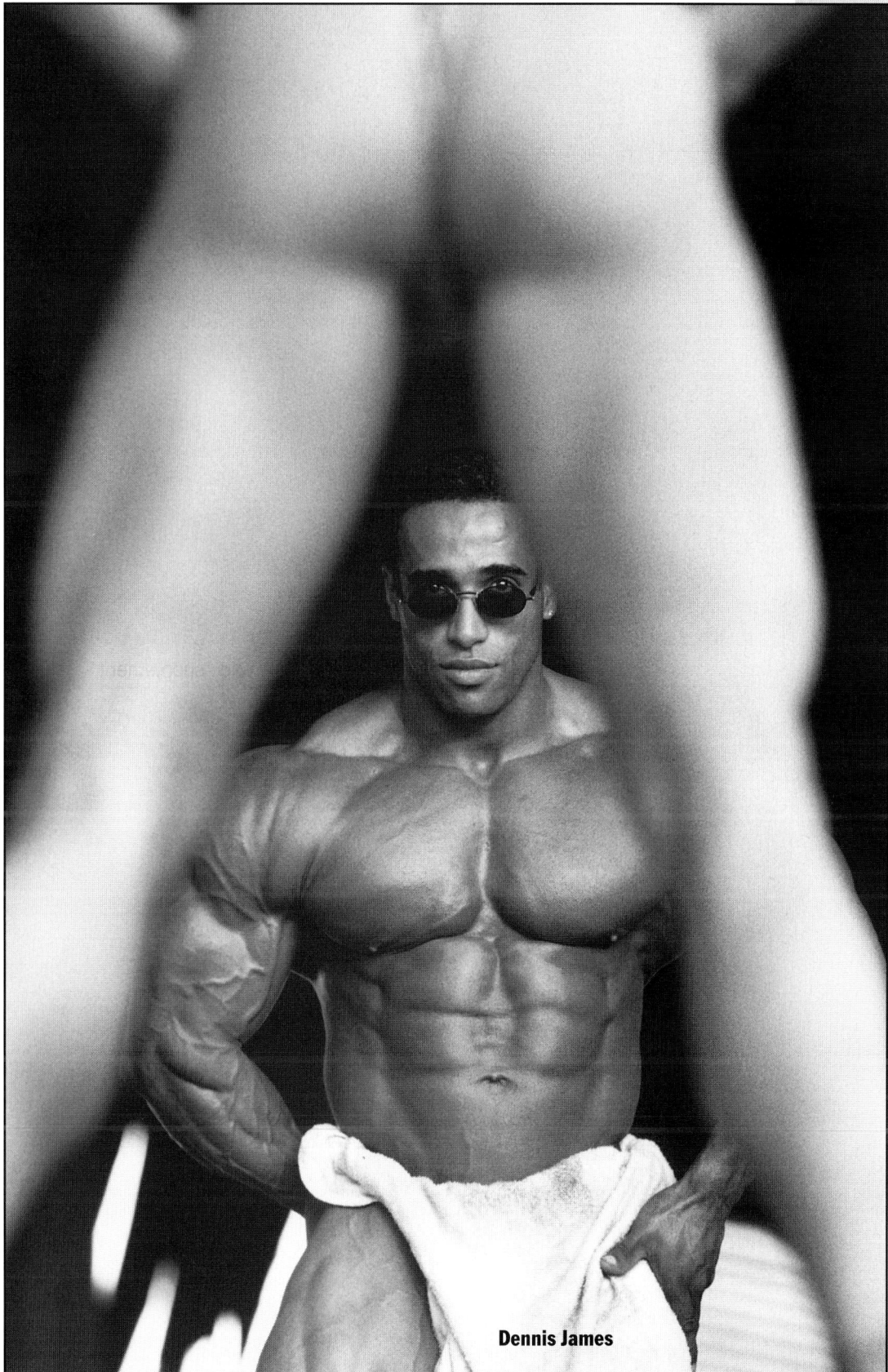

Dennis James

CHAPTER EIGHT

Glutamine

Glutamine is one of the next generation of supplements that is revolutionizing natural bodybuilding. Along with creatine, it is setting the standard for all future supplements.

Glutamine is one of the most abundant non-essential amino acids in the human body, making up over 50 percent of amino acids found in muscle cells. Please don't let the word non-essential mislead you. Even though the body can manufacture glutamine from other sources (thus meeting the definition of non-essential), in times of stress (exercise, for example) glutamine levels may drop dangerously low.[2] The end result is the aspiring bodybuilder's worst nightmare – negative nitrogen balance leading to muscle wasting. High levels of glutamine counteract this by keeping the body in positive nitrogen balance – the necessary environment for laying down new muscle tissue.[1]

Besides its role in preventing muscle wasting, glutamine stimulates the activity of immunocytes – small cells that can be called the garbage collectors of the body. Among their functions is the tracking down and removal of metabolism waste products. The faster the waste products are removed, the faster muscle recovery takes place. As an example, in one study athletes receiving glutamine had half as many infections following intense exercise as non-using athletes.[5]

Not convinced yet? There's more. Depending on glycogen levels, glutamine can be converted into glutamate, and then into the amino acid alanine. Big deal you say. Well it just so happens that the liver can convert alanine into glucose, which is then returned to the muscles to be used as an energy source. The process is just one example of what biochemists call gluconeogenesis – the production of glucose from nonglucose sources.

Other important functions of glutamine include:
1) stimulation of the immunity system
2) structural integrity of various organs
3) fuel source for red and white blood cells
4) role in the molecular process of transcription

Finally, glutamine supplementation helps muscle cells maintain maximum volume by preserving their most abundant amino acids, taurine and glutamine. Clinical studies have consistently demonstrated the role of these amino acids in muscle growth, protein synthesis and antiprotolysis (inhibition of protein catabolism). If glutamine and taurine levels drop below a certain point, protein synthesis stops. This means zero progress, and no muscle growth.

Now hold on just a minute. You're probably saying, "I take creatine, and it's done wonders for my workouts. Why would I need glutamine?" Creatine primarily contributes to your energy reserves, while glutamine plays a large role in muscle tissue regeneration. The two naturally go together.

Remember that lifting weights is necessary to stimulate muscle growth, but that chronic exercise stress results in the paradoxical decrease in plasma testosterone and growth hormone levels.[3] Glutamine has been shown to significantly elevate growth hormone levels.[4] Instead of spending a fortune on HGH (and the risks that go with it), glutamine stimulates your own GH levels to the max.

HOW MUCH?

Although the scientific literature recommends five to 10 grams per day, the volume of anecdotal evidence from bodybuilders suggests 10 to 20 grams of glutamine per day. And, like creatine, it probably makes more sense to take four, five-gram dosages throughout the day, rather than taking the full 20 grams at once. Not only does this insure better absorption, but also, for many people, the higher concentration may be hard on the gastrointestinal tract. Like most of the natural supplements discussed in this book, stick with a reputable brand like EAS, Twin Lab or the latest version released by Robert Kennedy, Formula One glutamine.

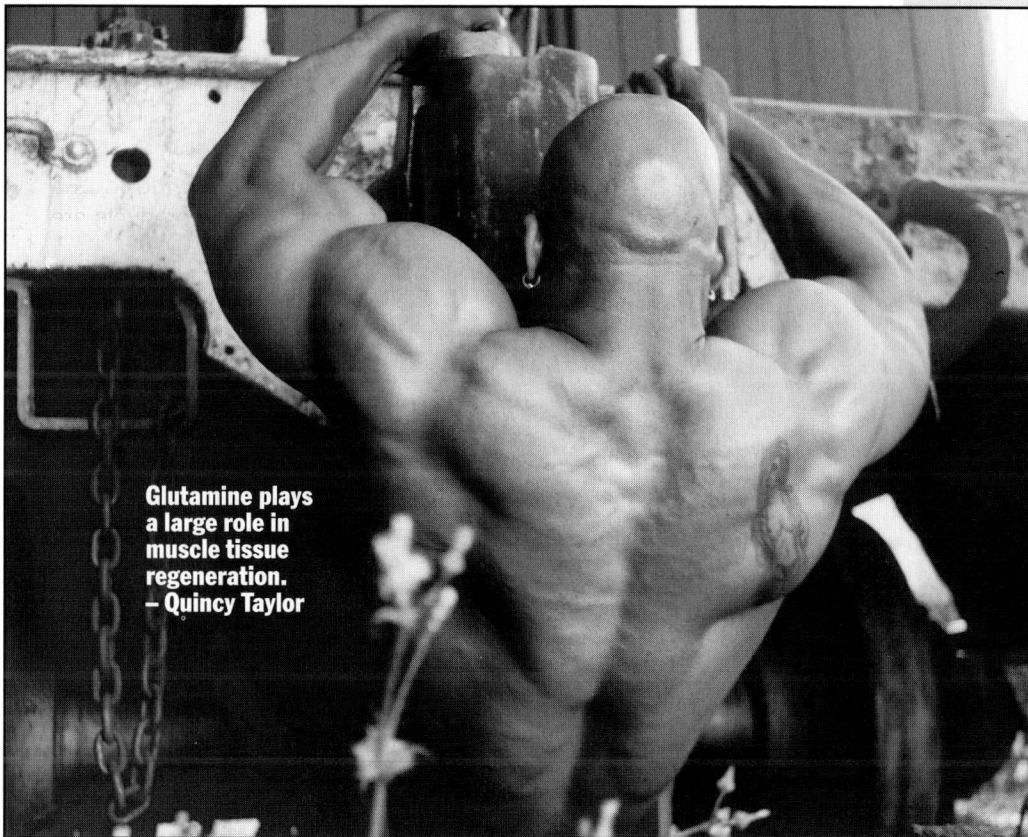

Glutamine plays
a large role in
muscle tissue
regeneration.
– Quincy Taylor

References
1) Keast, D., et al. Depression of plasma glutamine concentration after exercise stress and its possible influence on the immune system. *Medical Journal of Australia*, 162: 1995, 15-18.
2) Lacey, J.M., Wilmore, D.W. Is Glutamine a conditionally essential amino acid? *Nutrition Reviews*, 48: 1990, 297-309.
3) Rowbottom, D.G. et al. The emerging role of glutamine as an indicator of exercise stress and overtraining. *Sports Medicine*, 21: 1996, 80-97.
4) *Neuroendocrinology*, 57 (6): 1993, 985-990.
5) Rohde, T., et al. Glutamine, exercise, and the immune system: Is there a link? *Exercise Immunology Review*, 4, 49-63, 1998.

CHAPTER NINE

Hydroxy Methylbutyrate – HMB

In the early 1980s researchers at Iowa State University discovered that HMB, a metabolite of the amino acid leucine, played a major role in protein metabolism. Researchers theorized that HMB decreased protein catabolism by interfering with the enzymes responsible for protein breakdown.[1]

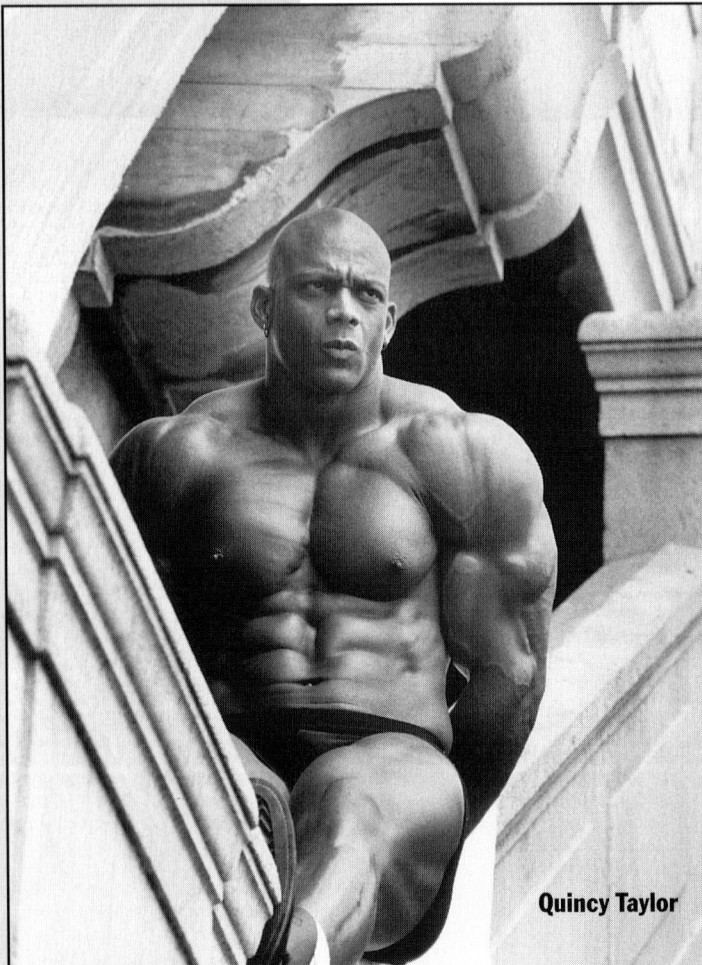

Quincy Taylor

HMB is similar to creatine in that it has good scientific research to back it up. Research with human subjects has shown significant increases in muscle mass and strength. In one well documented study, 41 untrained subjects were divided into three groups; with one group receiving a placebo (inactive substance), and the two others receiving 1.5 or three grams of HMB per day. After a four week resistance program, those receiving the HMB showed significant increases in muscle mass and strength, and decreased levels of such catabolic indicators such as creatine phophokinase and 3-methyl histidine.[2] Another study compared HMB on trained and untrained subjects using three grams per day of the supplement. When tested on a one-rep maximum bench press, the trained group had significant increases in strength, and decreased levels of bodyfat.[3]

HMB got its first big break in bodybuilding from *MuscleMedia* magazine publisher Bill Phillips. He began marketing the supplement in the mid-1990s under the banner of his company, EAS. In many respects Bill took a gamble, as up to that time few peer-

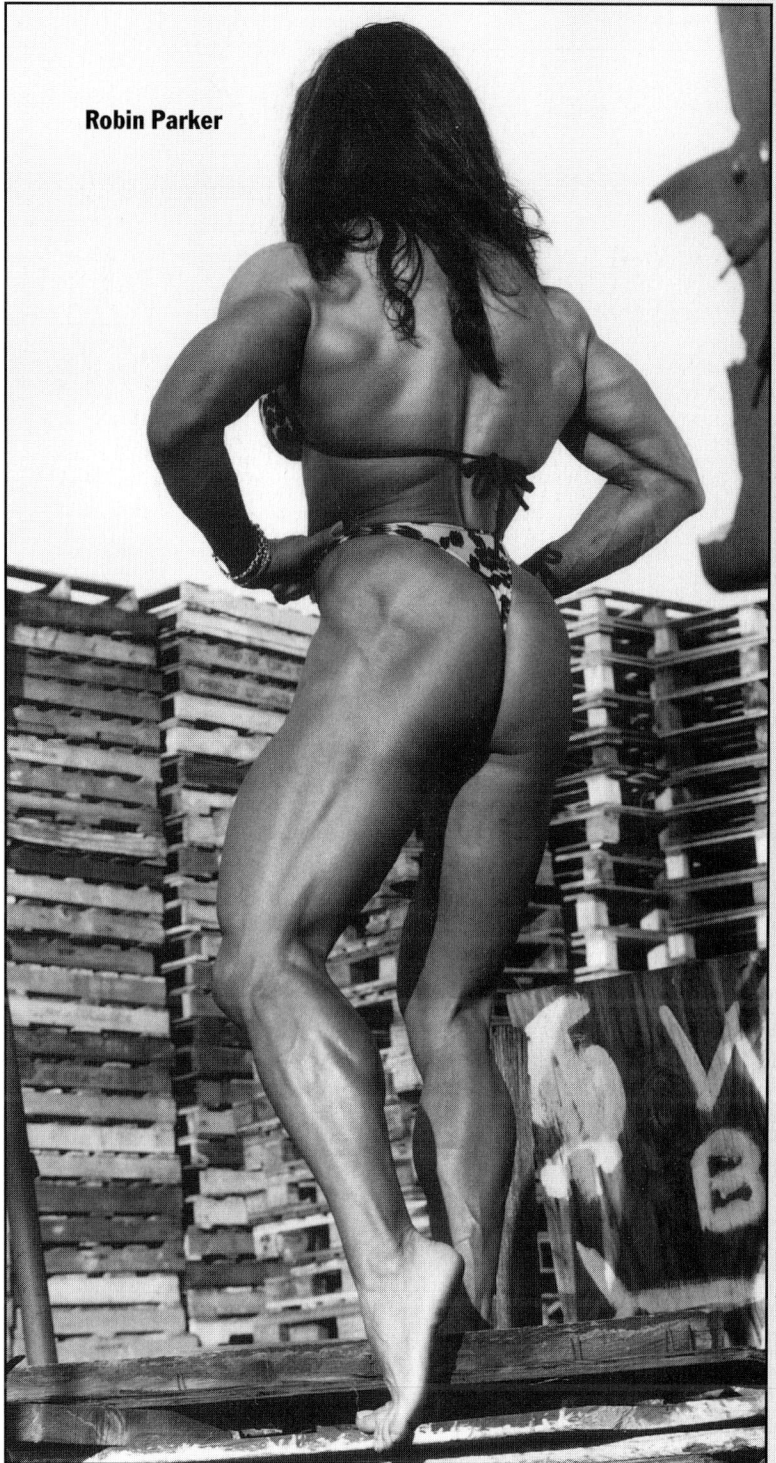

reviewed studies on HMB had been conducted. Competitors were quick to criticize Phillips for this, but research started to back up his claims, and now most of the rivals have come out with their own version of HMB.

DOSAGE

Studies with HMB have suggested three to five grams per day is the optimum dosage. Of course bodybuilders tend to take more, but then the issue of cost comes into play. HMB is one of the more costly supplements available. A top brand quality product can set you back $100 to $120 a month. Your best option is probably to cycle HMB with another quality supplement, like glutamine or creatine. Cycling means to alternate one substance with another. For example, you could take glutamine for four to six weeks, and then switch to HMB or creatine. Not only is this easier on the pocket book, but cycling helps prevent the development of tolerance that usually occurs after long-term use of a supplement.

As of winter 1999, there were no reported side effects associated with light to moderate (one to five grams per day) HMB use. Of course, like creatine, HMB is such a new supplement that there are no long-term studies to refer to. Still, the fact that HMB is a naturally occurring metabolite, should mean that it's relatively safe provided it's not abused (i.e. heavy dosages for extended periods of time).

Robin Parker

References

1) Armsey, T.D., Green, G. Nutrition supplements: Science versus hype. *The Physician and Sports Medicine*, 25 (6) 1997, 76-92.

2) Nissen, S.L., et al. The effect of the leucine metabolite HMB on muscle metabolism during resistance exercise training. *Journal of Applied Physiology*, 81 (5) 2095-2104, 1996.

3) Nissen, S.L., et al. The effect of HMB supplementation on strength and body composition of trained and untrained males undergoing intense resistance training. 10 (3), 287, 1996.

CHAPTER TEN

Gamma Hydroxybutyrate (GHB) and Substitutes

GHB is one of those supplements that had a couple of good years and then faded away. True, it's still being used as an entertainment drug, and a few perverts use is as a date rape drug, but in athletic circles it's all but forgotten.

GHB is a compound found mainly in the hypothalamus of the brain. In many respects it fits the criteria of a neurotransmitter (brain messenger). GHB received its first big boost in the late 1980s when Japanese researchers found that test subjects receiving 2.5 grams of GHB had their growth hormone levels elevated by up to 16 times the normal rate. What made the tests alluring to athletes was that none of the test subjects were growth hormone deficient to begin with. It's one thing for a supplement to boost hormone levels back to normal, but something else if it can boost them above normal.

As would be expected, the relationship between GHB and growth hormone was seized on by supplement manufacturers. They promoted GHB as a cure for everything from impotence to old age. Unfortunately, as later studies found, the elevated growth hormone levels had little effect on muscle size or strength. In fact elevated growth hormone levels are quickly followed by decreased levels. From a bodybuilding point of view, GHB is a supplement dead end. It would be nice if this was the end of the story, but it's not.

GHB – DOWN AND DIRTY

In recent years, GHB has received a lot of attention – not on the playing field, but in the bedroom! Although limited, the evidence suggests GHB can boost sexual responsiveness and sleep. (A contradiction if there ever was one.)

The most popular theory for GHBs mechanism of action is that it blocks the uptake of the brain transmitter dopamine. The less dopamine removed, the more pronounced its effects. Within 60 minutes of ingesting GHB most individuals go into a deep sleep. In theory, GHB should make a good anesthetic, but its effects only last for two to four hours. Now, while having little application for surgery, the drugs powerful sedative effects have been latched onto by a few demented individuals for use as a date rape agent. Whether the victim passes out or remains semi-conscious, the end result is the same – sexual violation with little or no memory of the attack.

Besides inducing sleep, GHB supposedly enhances sexual perfor-mance. As might be expected, there's not a lot of scientific evidence to back this up. Virtually everything is based on anecdotal reports. The problem with this should be obvious. Who is going to say his or her performance was lacking? We strongly advise a healthy dose of skep-ticism when evaluating such reports. In fact, hopefully the next paragraph will turn you away for good.

THE SILENT KILLER

On the surface any drug that can boost sexual performance or induce sleep sounds like a god send. Unfortunately, GHB can also be a killer. A couple of bodybuilders have died after slipping into a GHB-induced coma. Granted

> GHB can depress the ANS to fatal levels.
> – Hamdullah Aykutlu

alcohol and other drugs were also involved, but the fact remains that GHB can depress the autonomic nervous system (ANS) to fatal levels.

A FINAL WORD FOR BASEMENT CHEMISTS

Thanks to that great 90s phenomenon – the internet – making your own GHB is now an option. You can download a complete recipe; complete with ingredients to concoct GHB in your own kitchen. As great as this sounds in theory, we strongly advise against it. We're not going to repeat our list of reasons against such foolhardiness, they can be found in *Anabolic Primer*. Suffice to say making your own GHB could put you to sleep permanently.

GHB SUBSTITUTES

The decline of GHB as an athletic drug has led to the search for other related substances that will boost performance without GHB's negative attributes. The following are two such examples:

1,3-BD (1,3 butanediol or 1,3 butylene glycol)

Consumption of 1,3-BD decreases appetite, and the storage of bodyfat. This drug has been added to animal feed to enhance metabolic stability in pigs, reduce infant mortality and raise the blood sugar and liver glycogen levels of offspring when fed to the mother late in pregnancy. It has also been

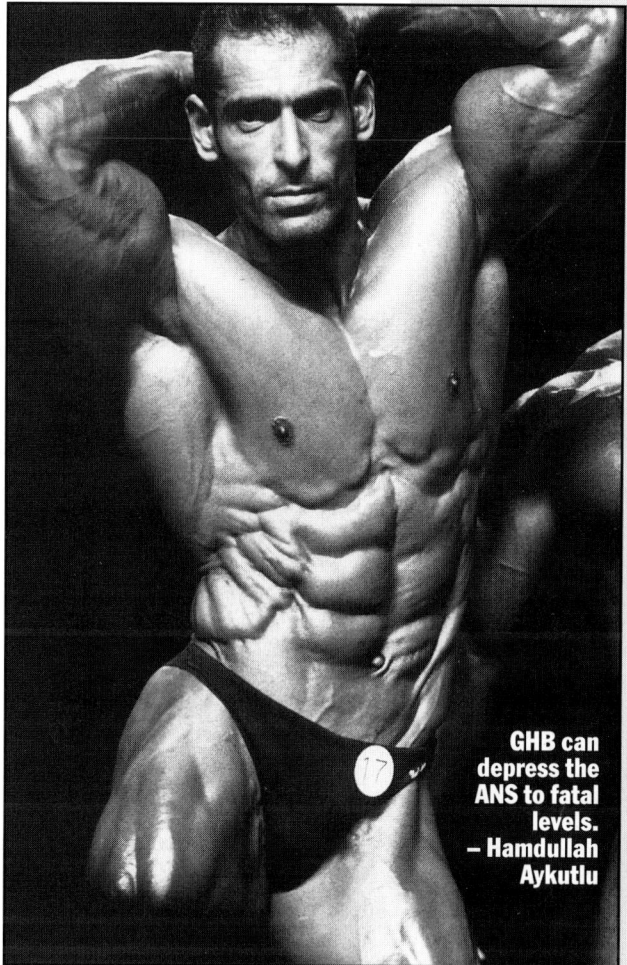

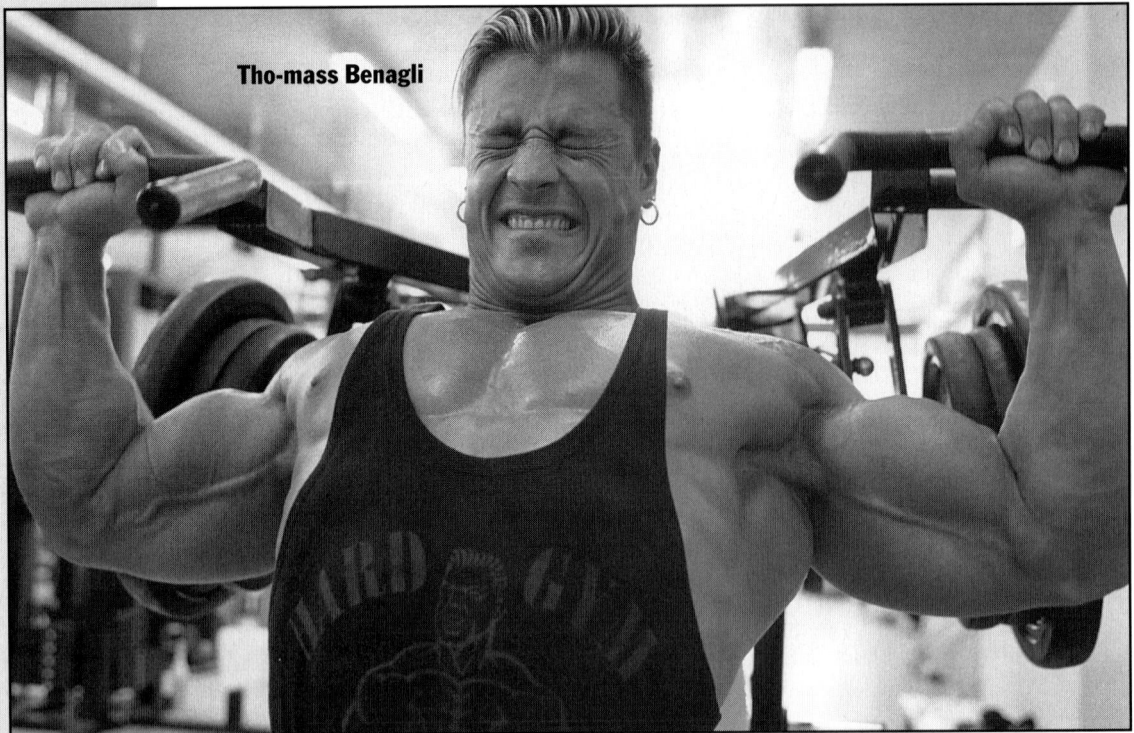

Tho-mass Benagli

used to treat hypoglycemia in turkeys. This drug also has potent post-stroke potential. It has been shown to prevent or minimize damage to the brain in oxygen deprived mice. Two more advantages of 1,3-BD are: it is a topical agent used to treat balding, and it does not posses the psychoactive properties of GHB. For ergogenic purposes, it is believed to improve strength and energy, while reducing bodyfat levels.

1,4-BD (tetramethylene 1,4-diol or 1,4 butylene glycol)

Found naturally in plants, 1,4-BD has many medicinal properties including: anti-oxidant, antibacterial, antitumor-forming, antiviral, anti-inflammatory, antiallergic, HIV inhibiting, immune modulating, white blood cell mobilizing, cardiotonic, antiasthmatic, antimalarial, ulcer inhibiting and increasing brain dopamine levels. It is, therefore, considered to be an antiaging drug. Long-term usage (over six months) in animals found that 1,4-BD acted as a sex hormone moderator and antagoniser. It is converted into GHB, which means it can increase GH production. This drug also eliminates the desire for alcohol. High doses of 1,4-BD can cause deep sleep and muscle spasms. It requires refridgeration.

Neither 1,4-BD or 1,3-BD are carcinogenic or toxic. A suggested regimen for bodybuilders is one gram of 1,3-BD, one hour before training; and one gram of 1,3-BD, with one gram of 1,4-BD, before bed. These drugs should be taken on an empty stomach, three hours after the last meal. This makes it a practical drug to use while training for a competition, but somewhat impractical for a bodybuilder who wishes to gain mass, and needs to eat more often.[1]

Reference
1) Angelidis. G. New Weapons For The Bodybuilders. *The Vault*, 24/7/97, Internet.

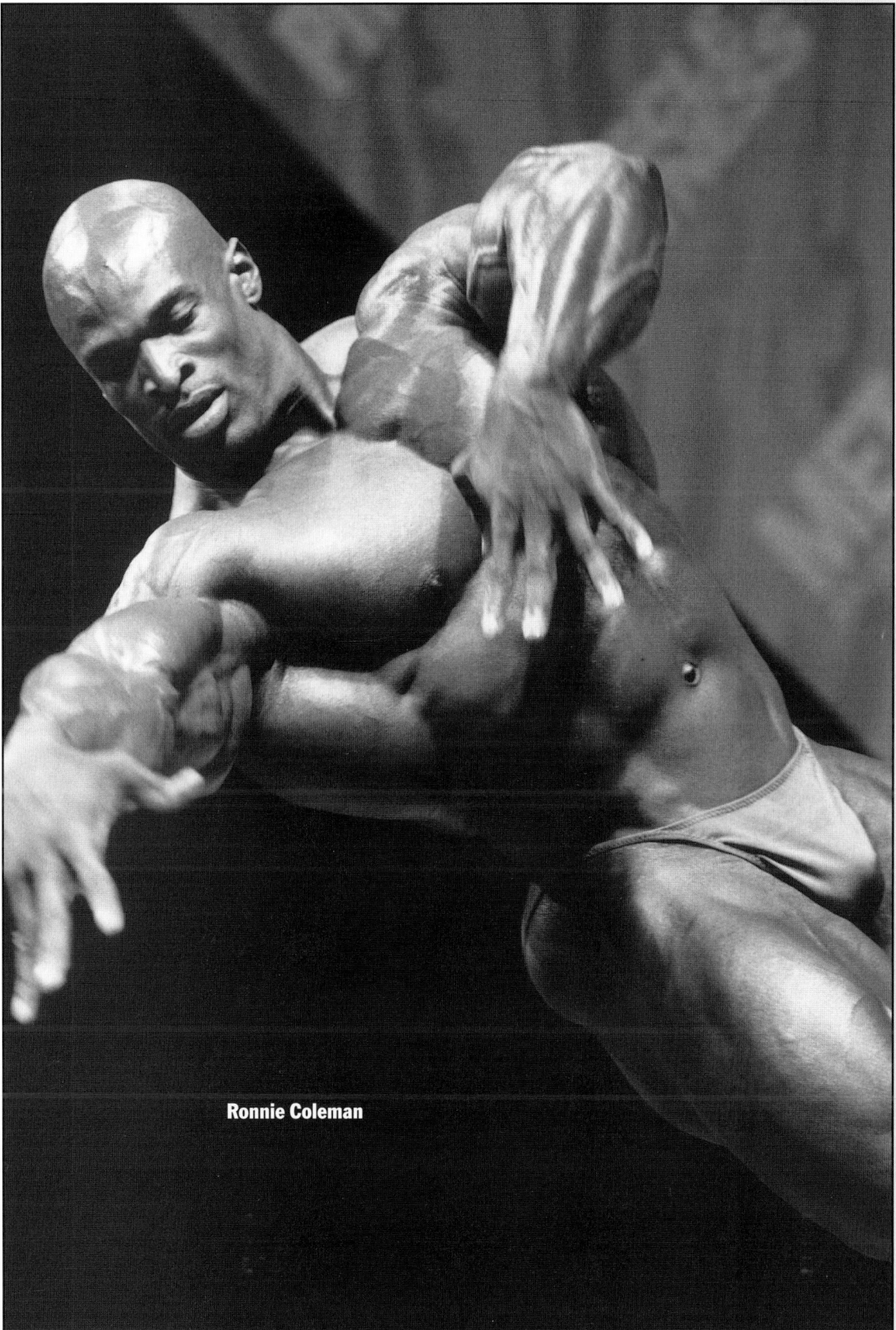

Ronnie Coleman

CHAPTER ELEVEN

Diuretics

Besides fat loss and muscle size, the third variable that competitive bodybuilders must control is water level. Even with fat levels down in the single digit percentage range, muscularity can still be hidden by a thin layer of water. The "smooth" look, it is often the difference between first and second place. When normal means fail to get rid of that last drop of water, bodybuilders (and many other athletes) turn to diuretics to obtain the ripped look.

WHAT THEY ARE

Diuretics are substances (both drugs and herbs) that assist the body in ridding itself of excess fluids, by increasing the rate of urine production by the kidneys. Many of the diuretics alter the excretion of electrolytes (these are chemicals that, when dissolved in a suitable solvent, can form a medium that will conduct an electric current), such as potassium and sodium salts. These two electrolytes are involved in numerous physio-logical processes including: muscle contraction, regulation of blood pressure and nerve impulse transmission.[4] Electrolytes themselves serve three general functions essential for survival. First, many are essential minerals. Second, they control the movement of water between body compartments. Third, they help maintain the acid-base balance required for normal cellular activities.

Electrolytes are dissolved in water, which can make up as much as 45 to 75 percent of total bodyweight. The concentration of solutes in the body fluids (which consist mostly of water) is the major determinant of fluid balance. Therefore, fluid balance implies electrolyte balance. If we alter one, we alter the other.[6] The results can

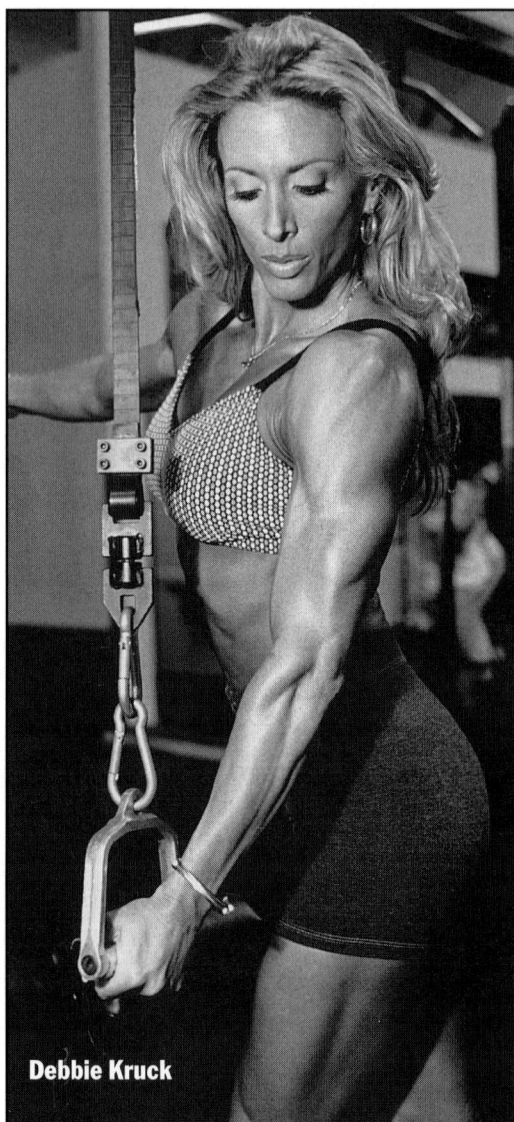

Debbie Kruck

be devastating. To remove excess water before a contest to show off ripped-muscles, bodybuilders take diuretics. But these drugs generally work by altering the electrolyte balance, in doing so they affect numerous metabolic systems, with fatal results. Never mind all the propaganda you've been fed about steroids, diuretics deserve every nasty comment and rumor that's made. These drugs serve an essential medical service, but without proper supervision, they can inflict pain, incapacitate, cause harm and kill. Diuretics are an unforgiving drug. Many require that you avoid certain foods and drugs. Do your homework, and if you do decide to try, get medical supervision. It's the only way to ensure you'll stay alive.

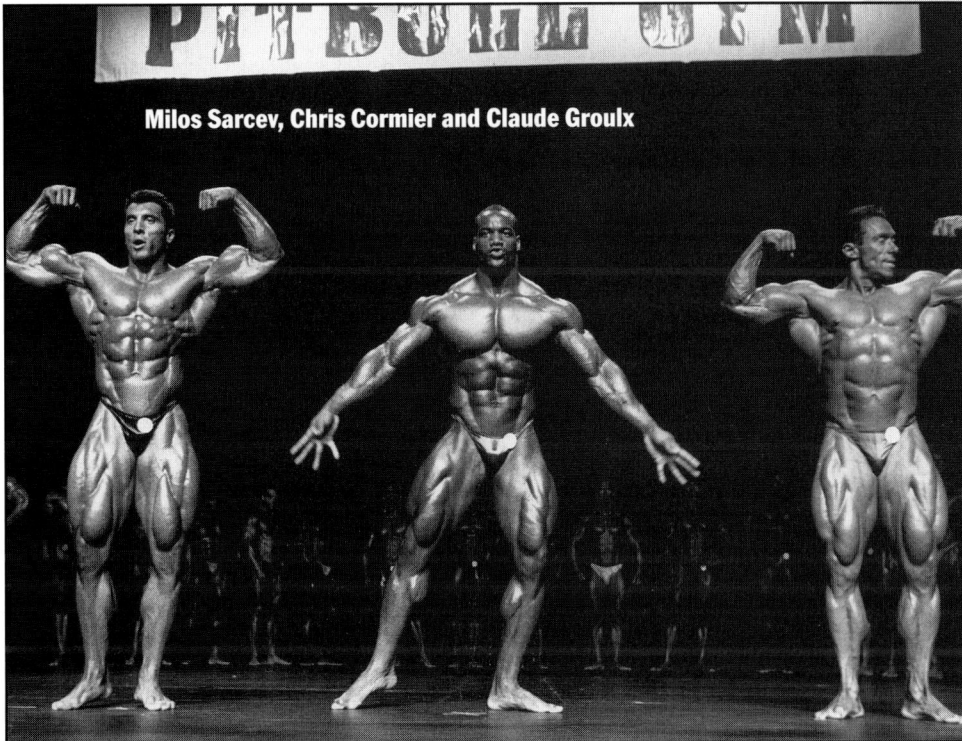

Milos Sarcev, Chris Cormier and Claude Groulx

WATER CONSERVATION IN THE HUMAN BODY

The body controls the amount of water excreted by hormonal control. Factors such as glomerular capillary pressure and blood volume act to regulate the amount of fluid initially absorbed by the kidney. The volume of urine excreted is controlled by the permeability (the ease at which a substance can cross a boundary) of the walls of specialized parts of the kidney called convoluted collecting tubules. This permeability is regulated by a hormone known as vasopressin, or antidiuretic hormone (ADH). In the absence of ADH, the water permeability of the distal convoluted tubule and collecting tubule is very low, and the final urine volume is correspondingly high. In the presence of ADH, water permeability is high, and the final volume is small. ADH has no effect on sodium absorption, but regulates the ability of water to osmotically follow ionic absorption.[5]

In addition, hormones called mineral corticoids help control electrolyte balance, particularly the concentrations of potassium and sodium. One of these, aldosterone, acts on the tubule cells in the kidneys, and causes

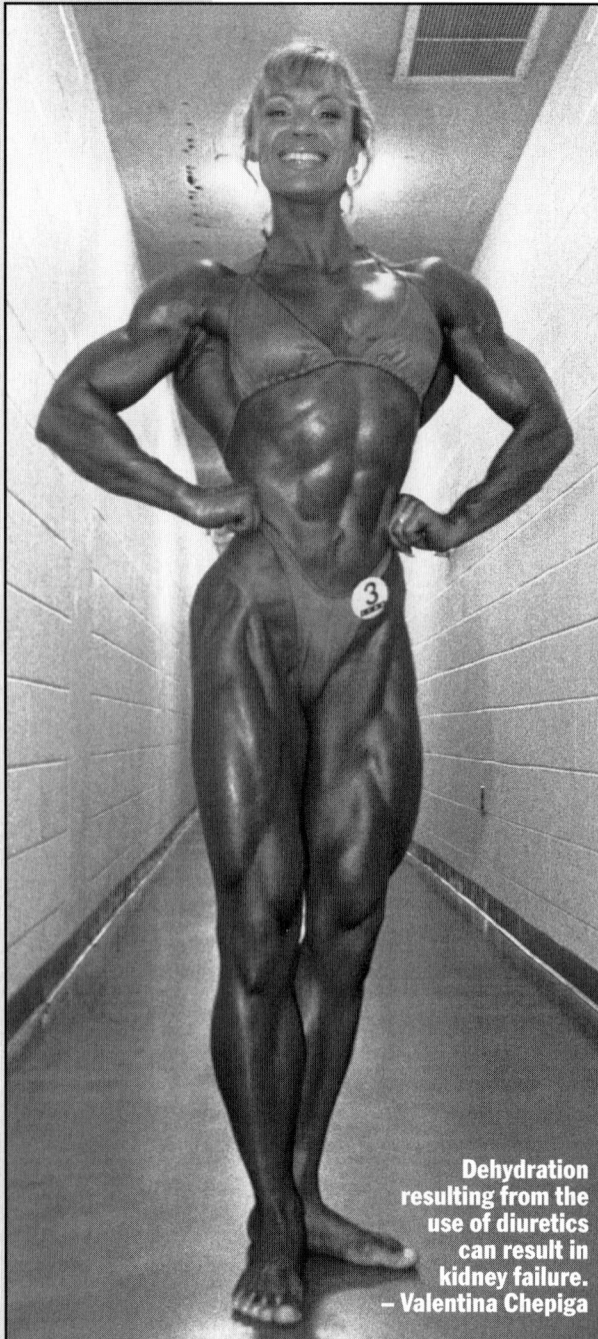

Dehydration resulting from the use of diuretics can result in kidney failure.
– Valentina Chepiga

them to increase their sodium reabsorption. As a result, sodium ions are removed from the urine and returned to the blood. In this manner, aldosterone prevents rapid depletion of sodium from the body. On the other hand, aldosterone decreases reabsorption of potassium. Large amounts of potassium are moved from the blood into the urine.

Conservation of sodium and excretion of potassium lead to a number of secondary effects. A large proportion of the sodium reabsorption occurs through an exchange reaction, whereby positive hydrogen ions pass into the urine to replace the positive sodium ions. The loss of hydrogen ions makes the blood less acidic and prevents acidosis. The movement of sodium ions also sets up a positively charged field in the blood vessels around the kidney tubules. As a result, negatively charged chloride and bicarbonate ions are drawn out of the urine and back into the blood. This increase in sodium-ion concentration in the blood vessels causes water to move by osmosis from the urine into the blood.[6]

The kidney, acting under both endocrine and neurologic control, has a primary role in coordination of electrolyte (primarily sodium) and water balance, between the external and internal environments. This part of the liquid portion of the blood consists of approximately 68,000 molecular weights. (Don't let this frighten you; it's just a measurement to compare the relative sizes of various molecules.) It is filtered through the capillary loops of the glomerulus. Then specialized blood vessels (afferent and efferent renal arterioles) act as variable resistors to maintain a relatively constant filtration pressure. If there is a decrease in aortic pressure, afferent arterioles constrict to help restore aortic pressure. This causes a decrease in renal blood flow. If a drug induces diuresis more rapidly than the blood can be rehydrated from the transcellular spaces, arterial hypotension occurs and afferent arterioles constrict.

Diuretics (with the exception of osmotic and water diuretics) exert their action by preventing establishment of a normal ion gradient by tubular cells. This interference with normal transport mechanisms, which principally move sodium back into the system from provisional urine, results in natriuresis. Since normal gradients are not established in tissues surrounding the loops of Henle, distal tubules and collecting ducts, water does not move out of provisional urine in normal quantities, and diuresis results. In as much as many edematous conditions are associated with a positive sodium balance, diuretics that interfere with sodium transport mechanisms are most effective in treatment of this class of edema.[2]

BODYBUILDING APPLICATIONS

Under strict medical supervision diuretics have important therapeutic applications in the elimination of excess fluid from body tissue in certain pathological conditions and for management of high blood pressure. Bodybuilders use diuretics for three reasons:

1) To reduce weight in order to drop to a lower-weight class.
2) Reduce water levels in the skin, to better reveal the musculature beneath.
3) If the competition is drug-tested, to reduce the concentration of prohibited substances by diluting the urine.

Unfortunately the rapid reduction in weight, and the severe dehydration that is the norm at the pro-level, can cause serious complications leading to kidney failure and death.[1]

WATER AS A DIURETIC

Consumption of water in excess of the homeostatic needs of the body will result in excretion of a large quantity of dilute urine. In many cases the body will shed so much water that water levels are actually lower than before the extra water consumption. As twisted as this may sound, you've actually used water to shed water! Thus in special cases, water can act like a diuretic.

OSMOTIC DIURETICS

Any significant increase in the amount of fluid in the body is usually accompanied by an increase in volume of urine voided. Sugars and sugar alcohols (i.e. glucose, sucrose, sorbitol and isosorbitol) may be used in medical settings for their osmotic diuretic effect. In general, the sugars must be given intravenously at high doses to produce diuresis.

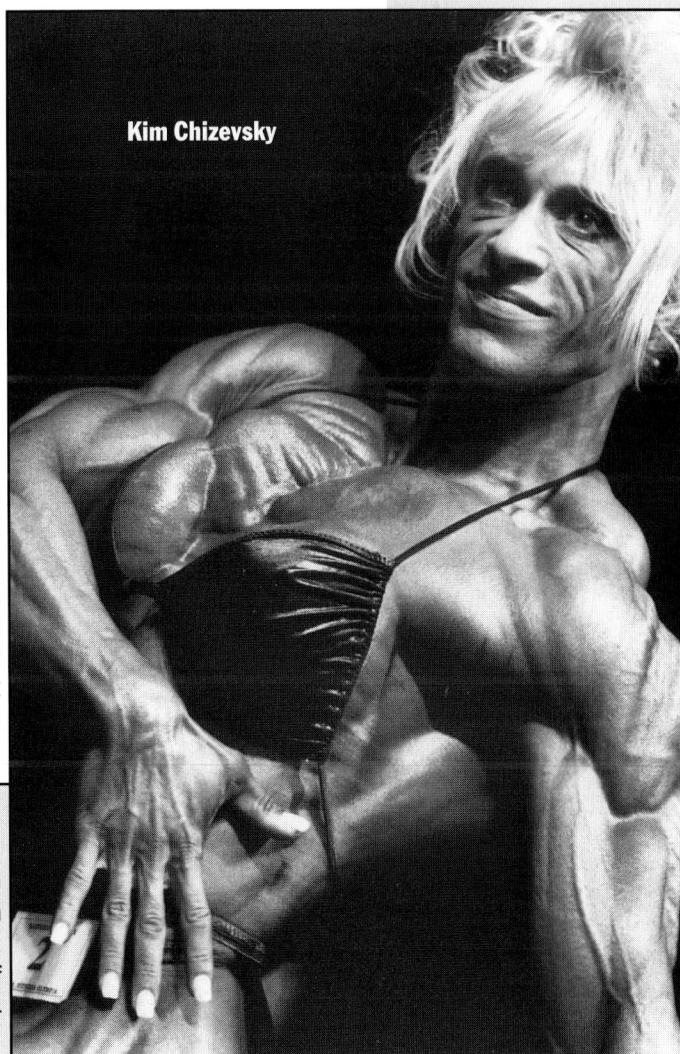

Kim Chizevsky

Trade Names: Osmitrol and Resectisol
Generic Name: Mannitol
Dosage: 50 ml ampules for I.V. injection as a 25 percent solution. Dose varies with the disease and renal response. Generally, the following dose is used: 1 to 2 mg/kg of a 5 to 10 percent solution at a rate of 4 ml/minute.[2]

MERCURIAL DIURETICS

These drugs are pH dependent and appear to act by liberation of a small amount of mercuric ion. This combines with cysteine, found in enzymes associated with transport systems located in the proximal and beginning distal tubules. Misuse of mercurial diuretics can cause acute renal insufficiency, that may be temporary or permanent.[2]

Trade Name: Novasurol
Generic Name: Merbaphen
Dosage: Historic only, was used as an antisyphilitic agent[2]

Trade Name: Calomel
Generic Name: Mercurous Chloride
Dosage: Historic only, replaced by organic mercurials because of cathartic effects and uncertain intestinal absorption[2]

Trade Name: Salygran
Generic Name: Mersalyl
Dosage: 0.25 mg Hg/kg, i.m.[2]

Trade Name: Dicurin
Generic Name: Merethoxylline
Dosage: 0.25 mg Hg/kg, i.m.[2]

Trade Name: Thiomerin
Generic Name: Mercaptomerin Sodium
Dosage: 0.25 mg Hg/kg, i.m. or subcutaneously (s.c.)[2]

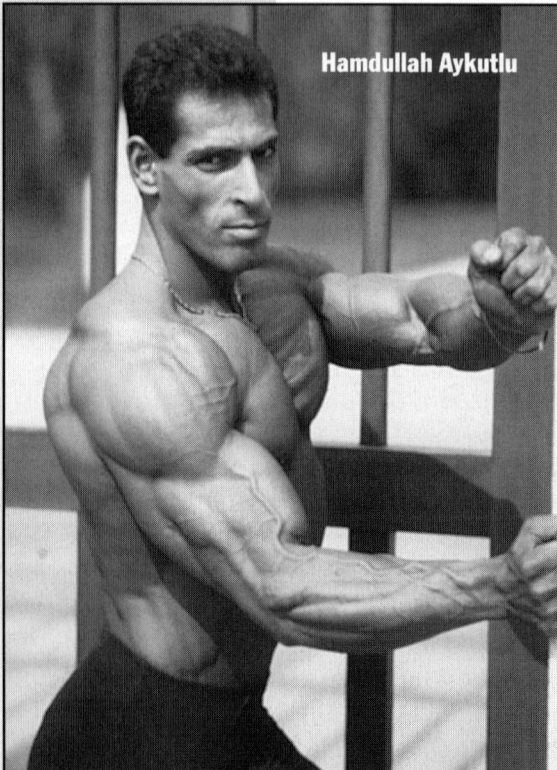

Hamdullah Aykutlu

CARBONIC ANHYDRASE INHIBITORS

Transport mechanisms that exchange potassium and sodium ions, in urine, for excess hydrogen ions, in extracellular fluid, exist in many locations along the renal tubular system. Hydrogen ions become available for this exchange, in the presence of carbonic anhydrase (an enzyme), by conversion of carbon dioxide and water to carbonic acid. Carbonic anhydrase is present in large concentrations, especially in tubular epithelial cells. Drugs that inhibit carbonic anhydrase will inhibit ion exchange mechanisms; causing sodium retention, and a preferential exchange of potassium ions for sodium (that are recovered from urine). An isosmotic quantity of water is excreted with the increased levels of sodium and potassium ions. The diuretic effect of these agents is lost after a few days, since in that time enough hydrogen ion accumulates to allow the exchange process to proceed. The main therapeutic uses of carbonic anhydrase inhibitors are treatment of chronic glaucoma and udder edema.[2]

Trade Name: Diamox
Generic Name: Acetazolamide
Dosage: 1 to 3 mg/kg/day, orally
        1 mg/kg/day, i.m.
        2 to 4 mg/kg/day, orally[2]

Trade Name: Daranide
Generic Name: Dichlorphenamide
Dosage: 2 to 4 mg/kg/day, orally[2]

Trade Name: Neptazane
Generic Name: Methazolamide
Dosage: 2 to 4 mg/kg/day, orally[2]

Trade Names: Cardrase and Ethamide
Generic Name: Ethoxzolamide
Dosage: 2 to 15 mg/kg/day, orally in divided doses[2]

BENZOTHIADIAZIDES (THIAZIDES)

These drugs exert their effect primarily on the proximal tubule, to prevent reabsorption of sodium. Some of the thiazides directly influence water reabsorption, perhaps through carbonic anhydrase inhibition. These drugs work close to the site of aldosterone-stimulated sodium-potassium exchange. A possible side effect of their use is excessive potassium loss in the presence of high aldosterone activity, as seen in congestive heart failure. Thiazides have some diabetogenic effects, especially in cases of diabetes mellitus.

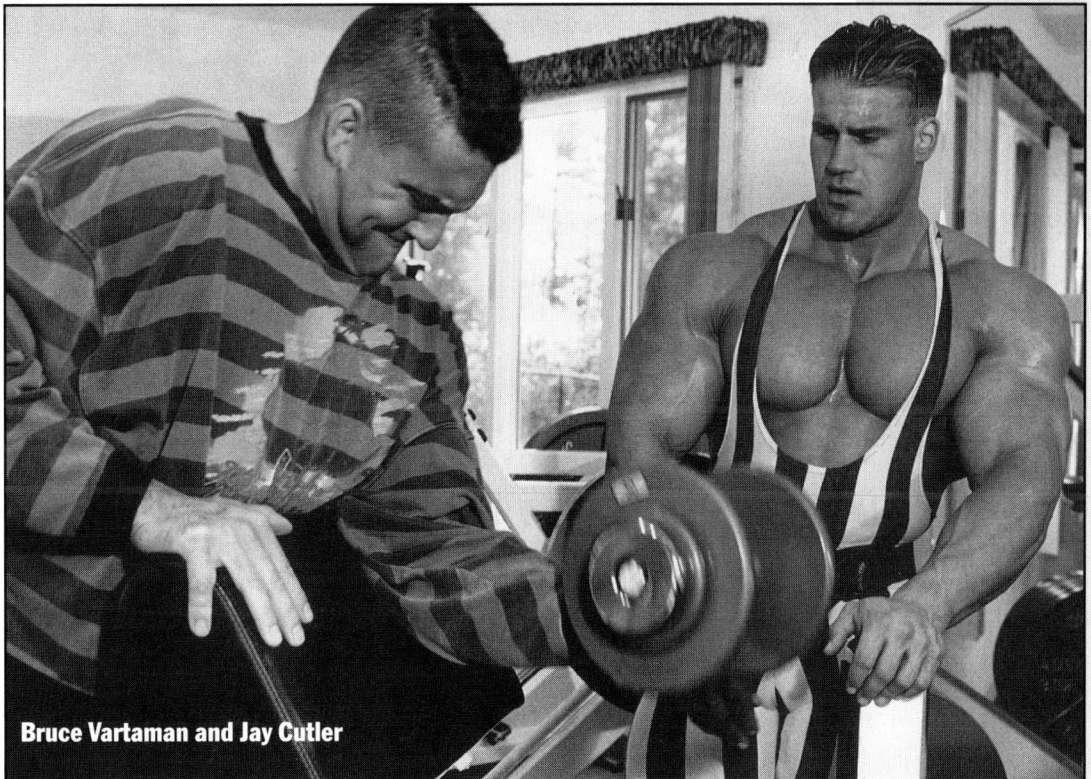

Bruce Vartaman and Jay Cutler

Use of these drugs can lead to loss of iron in the urine and inflammation of the pancreas.[2] The main therapeutic uses of these drugs are management of edema (swelling), associated with congestive heart failure and diabetes.

Trade Name: Diuracil
Generic Name: Chlorothiazide
Dosage: 12 to 15 mg/kg, orally

Trade Names: Hydrodiuril, Dyazide, Esidrix and Oretic
Generic Name: Hydrochlorothiazide
Dosage: 1 mg/kg, i.v.

Trade Name: Saluron
Generic Name: Hydroflumethiazide
Dosage: 1 mg/kg, orally

Trade Names: Aquatag and Edemex
Generic Name: Benzthiazide
Dosage: 0.10 to 0.15 mg/kg, orally

Trade Name: Naqua
Generic Name: Trichlormethiazide
Dosage: 0.10 to 0.15 mg/kg, orally

Trade Name: Enduron
Generic Name: Methylclothiazide
Dosage: 0.10 to 0.15 mg/kg, orally

Trade Names: Anhydron and Fluidil
Generic Name: Cyclothiazide
Dosage: 0.10 to 0.15 mg/kg, orally

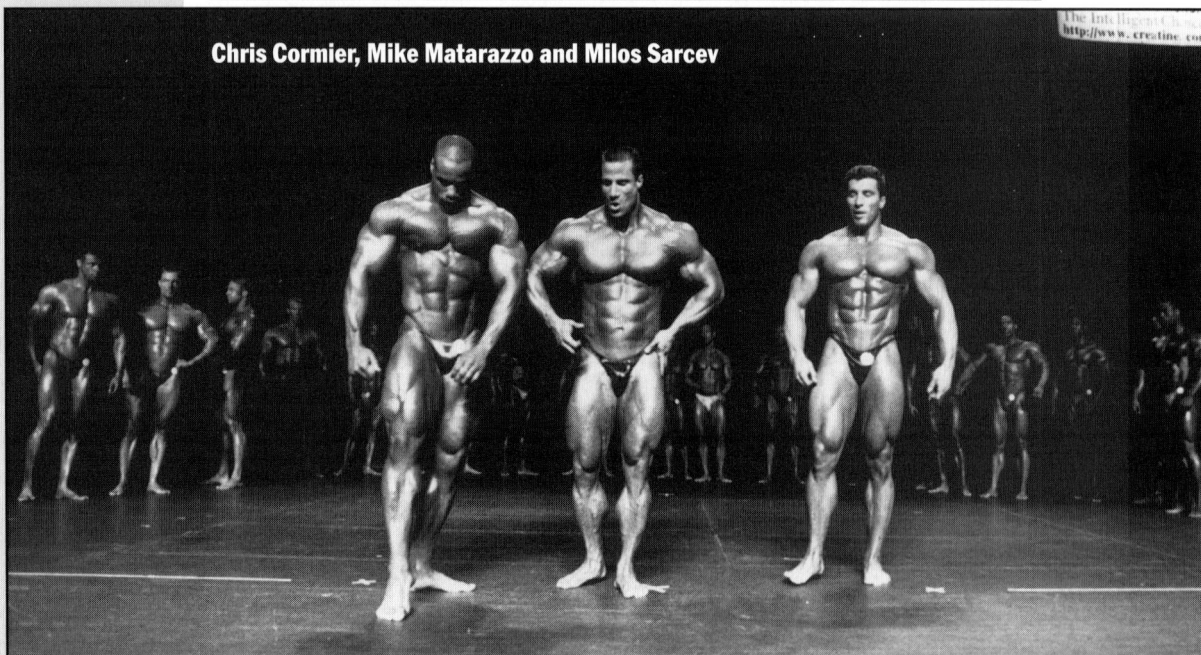

Chris Cormier, Mike Matarazzo and Milos Sarcev

ALDOSTERONE ANTAGONISTS

The body's primary hormone responsible for conserving water is aldosterone. Some of the most powerful diuretics available work by interfering with the actions of aldosterone; hence they are called aldosterone antagonists.

> Trade Name: Aldactone
> Generic Name: Spironolactone
> Dosage: 0.5 to 1.5 mg/kg alone or in combination with a thiazide or other diuretic.
> Thiazides cause potassium excretion, which is mainly the result of exchange of sodium for potassium in the distal tubule, an exchange that is almost entirely under the control of aldosterone. Since potassium excretion is impeded by spironolactone, it is important that additional potassium be avoided in the diet. Increased serum potassium levels stimulate release of aldosterone, and the higher levels then stimulate potassium excretion. Spironolactone blocks the actions of aldosterone. Specifically, it stops the reabsorption of sodium in the proximal areas of the distal tubules of the nephrons; and prevents sodium reabsorption, by disabling enhancement of exchange mechanism with either potassium or hydrogen ions. Spironolactone may exert some estrogen-like activity.

POTASSIUM-RETAINING AGENTS

These drugs are believed to act directly on tubular transport of sodium. The effect appears to be independent of the plasma level of aldosterone. Nor are they inhibitors of carbonic anhydrase. The reduced rate of potassium excretion with these drugs has been attributed to inhibition of potassium secretion in the distal tubular network.

> Trade Name: Dyrenium
> Generic Name: Triamterene
> Dosage: 0.5 to 3 mg/kg, orally, 3 times daily
>
> Trade Name: Midamor
> Generic Name: Amiloride Hydrochloride
> Dosage: 1 mg/kg, i.v.

LOOP OF HENLE DIURETICS (LHDs)

These drugs affect reabsorption of sodium primarily in the ascending loop of Henle. The exact mechanism of action is unknown. LHDs do not inhibit carbonic anhydrase or affect aldosterone activity. They also exert action on the proximal and distal tubules. LHDs are readily absorbed from the GI tract. They only accumulate in the liver, where biliary excretion occurs. After I.V. injection, one third of the dose is excreted by the liver and two thirds by the kidneys. Elimination of LHDs is rapid enough so that accumulation of the drug does not occur with normal doses. These drugs are all potent diuretic-saluretics. If used excessively, they may result in dehydration and electrolyte imbalance. LHDs should not be used if potassium-depleting steroids are also being taken.

> Trade Name: Lasix
> Generic Name: Furosemide
> Dosage: 40 to 80 mg, 3 times daily, maximum daily dose 200 mg

Comments: This drug can have serious adverse effects. Since it is taken while dieting down for a contest, electrolyte depletion can result from decreased salt intake. The symptoms are: weakness, dizziness, drowsiness, poluria, polydipsia, orthostatic hypotension, lethargy, leg cramps, sweating, bladder spasms, anorexia, vomiting, mental confusion and meteorism (painful distension of the intestine with gas). The bloated abdomens sometimes seen on stage are often blamed on steroid use, but are more likely caused by the use of diuretics. Furosemide can also aggravate diabetes, and push borderline diabetics into full diabetes. Since many bodybuilders are also using insulin, anyone who chooses to use this drug should monitor his/her glucose levels closely.

> Trade Name: Edecrin
> Generic Name: Ethacrynic Acid, Ethacrynate Sodium
> Dosage: 40 to 80 mg, 3 times daily

Comments: Similar in potency to Furosemide, Ethacrynic Acid is a rapidly acting diuretic that may lead to excessive diuresis and natriuresis, with water depletion and electrolyte imbalance. An increase in salt intake and supplementary potassium chloride are often necessary with this drug. Among potential serious side effects: GI problems including nausea, vomiting and diarrhea (occasionally sudden and profuse severe diarrhea, which requires immediate discontinuance of the drug), vertigo and hearing loss.

To prevent rapid and excessive fluid and electrolyte losses, start with small doses. Onset of diuresis occurs at 50 to 100 milligrams, once achieved the minimally effective dose can be given on a continuous or intermittent schedule. The following schedule can be used to determine the minimum effective dose:

Day 1: 50 mg (single dose) after meal.
Day 2: 50 mg twice daily after meals.
Day 3: 100 mg in the morning, 50 to 100 mg after the evening meal (depending on the response to the morning dose).
Once the desired weight has been achieved, it is usually possible to reduce both the dosage and frequency of administration.

> Trade Names: Bumex, Burinex
> Generic Name: Bumetanide
> Dosage: 0.5 to 2 mg/day, further doses every 4 to 5 hours, for a maximum of 10mg/day

Comments: This drug is 40 times more potent than Furosemide. Excessive doses or too frequent administration can lead to: dehydration, electrolyte depletion, reduction in blood volume and circulatory collapse with a possibility of vascular thrombosis and embolism. This drug should not be used without medical supervision.

HERBAL DIURETICS

For those wanting to shed a little extra water, but not wanting to get involved with powerful diuretic drugs (a smart choice in our opinion), the following herbal substitutes are far safer.

Herbal diuretics belong to two groups: those that increase kidney blood flow and those that reduce water reabsorption in the nephrons of the kidney. Herbs that are cardio-active, and circulatory stimulants increase overall blood flow. The more blood passing through the kidneys, the more urine that is produced. Other herbs can change the osmotic balance, while being excreted by the kidneys, causing more water loss. The following is a list of diuretic herbs, with dosages. Most can be purchased at better health food stores. (All preparations are in one cup of hot water.)

Agrimony (Agrimonia eupatoria)
Dosage: 1 to 2 tsp, infuse 10 to 15 minutes, 3 times daily

Bearberry (Arctostaphylos uva-ursi)
Dosage: 1 to 2 tsp, infuse 10 to 15 minutes, 3 times daily

Blue Flag (Iris versicolor)
Dosage: 1 tsp, bring to a boil, then let simmer 10 to 15 minutes, 3 times daily

Boldo (Peumus boldo)
Dosage: 1 tsp, infuse 10 to 15 minutes, 3 times daily

Boneset (Eupatorium perfoliatum)
Dosage: 1 to 2 tsp, infuse for 15 minutes

Broom (Sarothamnus scoparius)
Dosage: 1 tsp, infuse for 10 to 15 minutes, 3 times daily

Buchu (Barosma betulina)
Dosage: 1 to 2 tsp, infuse for 10 minutes, 3 times daily

Bugleweed (Lycopus europaeus)
Dosage: 1 tsp, infuse 10 to 15 minutes, 3 times daily

Burdock (Arctium lappa)
Dosage: 1 tsp, infuse 10 to 15 minutes, 3 times daily

Celery Seed (Apium graveolens)
Dosage: 1 to 2 tsp, infuse 10 to 15 minutes, 3 times daily

Cleavers (Galium aparine)
Dosage: 2 to 3 tsp, infuse 10 to 15 minutes, 3 times daily

Corn Silk (Zea Mays)
Dosage: 2 tsp, infuse 10 to 15 minutes, 3 times daily

Elder (Sambucus nigra)
Dosage: 2 tsp, infuse 10 minutes, 3 times daily

Gravel Root (Eupatorium purpureum)
Dosage: 1 tsp, bring to a boil and let simmer 10 minutes, 3 times daily

Hawthorn (Crataegus spp.)
Dosage: 1 to 2 tsp dried berries as tea, drink regularly

Juniper (Juniperus communis)
Dosage: 1 tsp crushed berries, let steep 20 minutes, morning and night

Kola (Kola vera)
Dosage: 1 to 2 tsp powdered nuts, boil and simmer 10 to15 minutes, 3 times daily

Linden (Tilia europea)
Dosage: 1 tsp of blossoms, infuse 10 minutes, 3 times daily

Parsley (Petroselinum crispum)
Dosage: 2 tsp, infuse 5 to 10 minutes in a closed container, 3 times daily

Saw Palmetto (Serenoa serrulata)
Dosage: 1/2 to 1 tsp, boil and simmer for 5 minutes, 3 times daily

Stone Root (Collinsonia canadensis)
Dosage: 1 to 2 tsp, boil and simmer 10 to 15 minutes, 3 times daily

Wild Carrot (Daucus carola)
Dosage: 1 tsp of herb or 1/3 tsp of seeds, infuse 10 to 15 minutes, 3 times daily

Yarrow (Achillea millefolium)
Dosage: 1 to 2 tsp, 10 to 15 minutes, 3 times daily[4]

The following are diuretics that have been banned by the IOC.[1]

Trade Names: Diamox, AK-ZOL and Dazamide
Generic Name: Acetazolamide

Trade Name: Midamor
Generic Name: Amiloride

Trade Name: Naturetin
Generic Name: Bendroflumethiazide

Trade Names: Aquatag, Exna, Hyrex, Marazide and Proaqua
Generic Name: Benzthiamide

Trade Names: Aladiene, Aldactone (Germany),
Phanurane (France), and Soldactone (Switzerland).
Generic Name: Canrenone

Trade Name: Orimecur (Spain)
Generic Name: Chlormerodin

Trade Names: Hygroton, Hylidone and Thalitone
Generic Name: Chlortalidone

Trade Names: Daranide, Oratrol and Fenamide
Generic Name: Diclofenamide

Trade Names: Esidrix, Hydro-Diuril, Oretic and Thiuretic
Generic Name: Hydrochlorothiazide

Trade Name: Salygran
Generic Name: Mersalyl

Trade Names: Alatone and Aldactone
Generic Name: Spironolactone

Trade Name: Demadex
Generic Name: Torsemide

Trade Name: Dyrenium and Dyazide
Generic Name: Triamterene

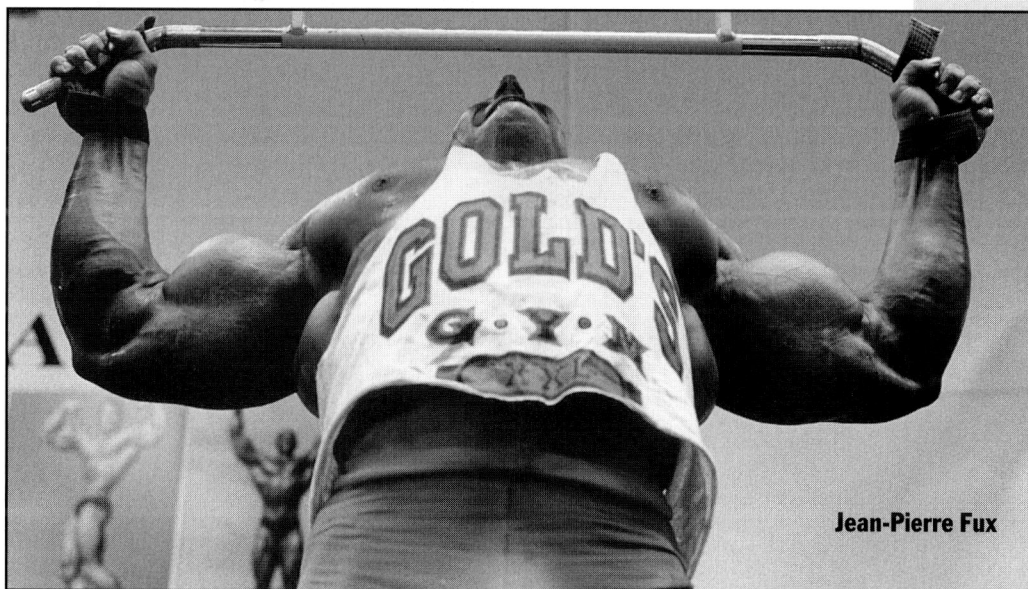

Jean-Pierre Fux

References
1) United States Olympic Committee, Diuretics. *Drug Control Education*,
   http:www.olympic-usa.org/inside/in.
2) Booth, N. and McDonald, L. (eds.). *Veterinary Pharmacology and Therapeutics*,
   6th edition, Iowa State University Press, Ames, 1988.
3) Krogh, C. (chief ed.). CPS, *Compendium of Pharmaceuticals and Specialties*,
   30th edition, Ottawa, Ontario, Canadian Pharmaceutical Association, 1995.
4) Hoffman, D. Diuretics, *Herbal Medicine*,
   http://www.healthy.net/library/books/hoffman/urinary/diuretics.htm.
5) Fogiel, M. (director of REA). *The Biology Problem Solver*,
   Research And Education Association, New York, 1984.
6) Tortora, G. and Anagnostakos, N. *Principles of Anatomy and Physiology*,
   2nd edition, Harper & Row, New York, 1978.

CHAPTER TWELVE

Good Blood, Bad Blood

In a manner of speaking just about every substance we discuss in this book has some impact on the blood stream – the body's transport highway. But we felt it necessary to include a separate chapter dealing with a few substances that athletes use to directly modify their circulatory systems. The use of buffering agents is legal, and not banned by sports' organizations, but has limited effectiveness. On the other hand, blood doping is very effective, but is banned by most sports organizations. Bodybuilders occasionally make use of buffering agents, while blood doping is primarily the technique of choice of aerobic athletes. Still we felt it necessary to discuss blood doping given the press it received at the 1998 Tour de France cycling race.[1]

BLOOD DOPING

From a medical point of view a blood transfusion is the intravenous administration of red blood cells (RBCs) or related blood products that contain RBCs. Such products can be obtained from blood drawn from oneself (autologous) or from a different person (heterologous). The most common indications for a blood transfusion in medicine are acute blood loss and severe anemia. The key point to remember is that blood transfusions take place when normal levels of RBCs are low.

Blood doping involves a transfusion of RBCs or erythropoietin (EPO, – a hormone released by the kidneys that increases RBC production) into individuals whose levels are normal. The primary function of RBCs is to transport oxygen; the more RBCs per unit area, the greater the oxygen carrying ability of the blood.

HOW IT'S DONE

The main technique for blood doping involves drawing out a liter of blood, freezing and storing it for a few weeks, and then reinfusing it. In theory this sounds straightforward, but there are hazards – chief of which is hygiene. Pathogens lurk around every corner just waiting for a chance to get into the body. Blood doping gives them three or four opportunities to invade the body. Most of the top athletes in the world have their own personal physicians helping in this practice. It's not something to be done in the kitchen and then stored in the family freezer.

Besides using blood, the second method of blood doping involves using erythropoietin (EPO). It is the body's primary hormone responsible for

"We are fed up with being treated like cattle. So we are going to behave like cattle...The sport is no longer interesting to anyone. We won't cycle and that's the end of it."

– Laurent Jalabert, the world's top-ranked cyclist, explaining the reasons behind a protest by cyclists in the 1998 Tour de France. Cyclists were upset by the media's focus on drug use in the sport.

RBC production. When RBC levels become low, EPO levels increase telling the various RBC manufacturing centers (i.e. spleen) to increase production.[2]

> Trade Name: Epogen
> Generic Name: Erythropoietin (EPO)
> Gym Dosage: 50 to 300 I.U./kg, i.v.

Comments: Since this drug improves endurance, it has little to no appeal for bodybuilders. Since EPO can increase RBC levels by as much as 40 percent, if aggravated by exercise-induced dehydration, this can lead to sludge-like blood, that can clog the arteries, leading to heart failure, stroke, pulmonary edema and death.[2] EPO is believed to be the cause of death among a number of elite Dutch cyclists. Users will start seeing effects in the second week of use. EPO should not be used for more than six weeks.[2]

EPOETIN

Epoetin is a genetically engineered copy of the hormone erythropoietin. It is used for treating severe anemia, cancer chemotherapy, AIDS patients and kidney dialysis patients. Athletes use it covertly for improved endurance and quicker recovery from strenuous exercise.

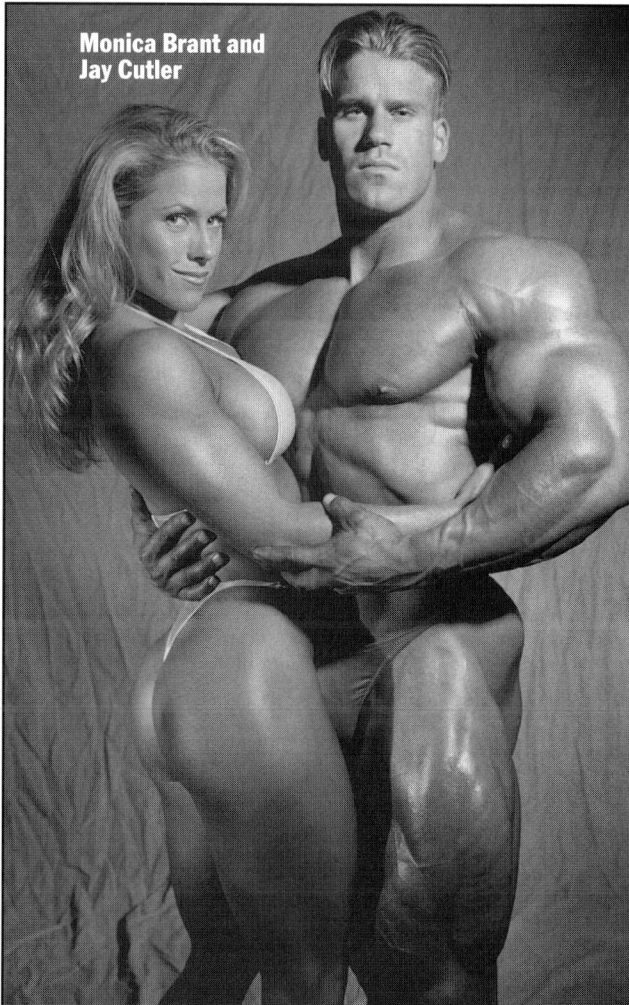

Monica Brant and Jay Cutler

WHERE THEY GET IT

Officially a carefully controlled prescription drug, but there's no control on the number of prescriptions written. Team doctors, who get a reported 10 percent of prize money from Tour de France teams, get EPO by prescription or on the black market, and can manipulate riders' red cell counts to be right at the legal limit for a race. Cycling officials allow a 50 percent level of red blood cells. Some riders admit to injecting themselves.

SIDE EFFECTS

As an athlete dehydrates, EPO can cause blood to thicken or clot, possibly causing strokes, kidney damage or heart attacks. Banned as a performance enhancer in sports. It is a health risk, but sports officials haven't approved an antidoping test for EPO.

Since the 1980s, 18 top European cyclists have died. Between 1989 and 1992, seven top orienteers died, including a 17-year-old female. In Holland

"Yes, I said I had taken EPO, how I took it and why I took it. I'm just a victim of a system...I felt like a criminal. Each rider had two police officers. They put me under pressure for four or five hours. They took everything. I undressed. They could see all of me. I went into a cell with a wooden bed... But I feel better inside because I have told the truth. Perhaps it is good for the sport."

– Competitor Armin Meir, member of the banned Festina Team, becoming the first Tour de France cyclist to admit taking the banned hormone, EPO.[1]

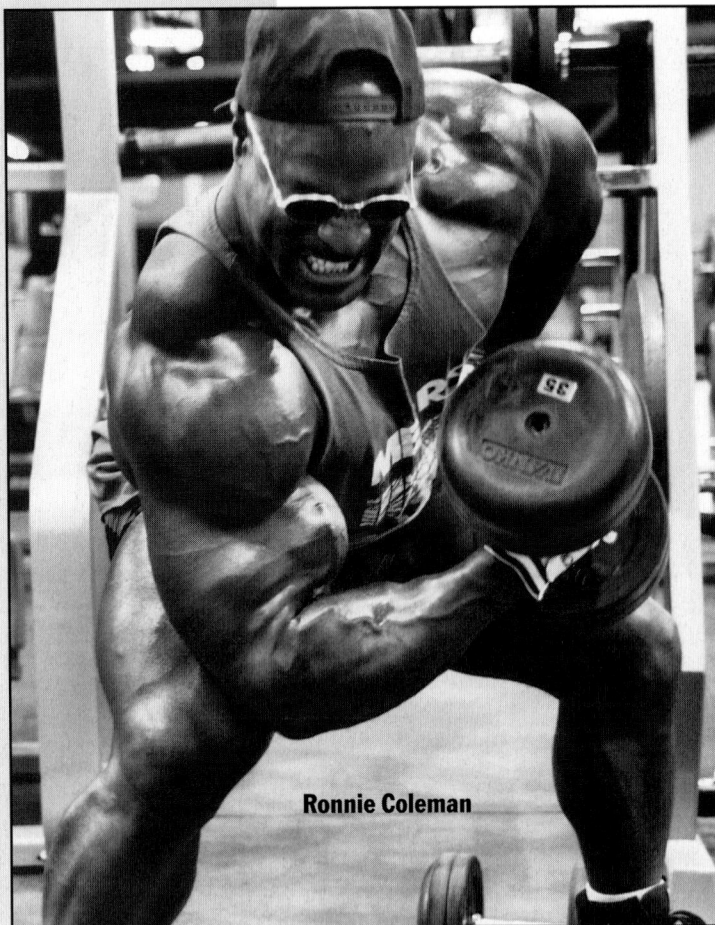

Ronnie Coleman

and Belgium, the two countries where the majority of the deaths occurred, investigation was scant.

"There weren't any EPO-related deaths here," commented Frans Stoele, a spokesman for the Netherlands Centre for Doping Affairs, in an interview. "In most cases people died of heart failure. One was a suicide. No autopsies were done because there was no suspicion about the cause of death." But North American scientists and heart specialists say it would be an incredible statistical aberration if most of the deaths were from natural causes.

"There's either been a massive cover-up (the investigations) or the people who did were massively incompetent. I think the cover-up is the likely answer," said Norman Gledhill, an exercise physiologist at York University in Toronto.[4]

TESTING

Within 10 hours, the hormones have disappeared from blood or urine, though their effects – in extra red blood cells, remain. For the past eight years, Raynald Gareau, a hematologist at the University of Quebec at Trois Rivieres, has been trying to find a test for EPO and other hormones favored by athletes. At last he has it. The latest results of his research project (a cooperative venture with scientists in Norway, France and Australia, will be published in January in *Medicine and Science in Sports and Exercise*. His test doesn't measure EPO directly. Instead, using blood samples drawn from athletes, he can find signs of unusual activity in the bone marrow, the body's factory for most blood cells. He measures the presence of a molecule, the soluble transferrin receptor, that scientists consider a marker of red blood cell production by the bone marrow.

The problem is the IOC, it does not accept such indirect markers of doping. Indirect markers are difficult to defend in court if an athlete challenges a punishment. Also, the IOC has chosen to test urine samples instead of blood.

The rules are outdated, Dr. Gareau said, and the IOC and other sports federations must change them if they hope to stop doping. The IOC held a special session on doping in February 1999, in Lausanne, Switzerland.

Even if Dr. Gareau's test does become standard in high-level athletics, he is not optimistic that he and other scientists will be able to keep ahead of the athletes. "If we are able to detect one kind of drug, the day after, or the week after, or the month after, another drug will probably arrive on the market."

DOING IT NATURALLY

One way to boost RBC levels naturally (courtesy of Mother Nature) has already been done by the US Olympic Team, with their Train Low/Live High system. At high altitude, oxygen levels are lower, and the body produces more erythropoietin to produce more RBCs to compensate. Olympic athletes are housed at these higher elevations. They are transported to lower elevations to train, and then returned to their accommodations in the mountains. Their increased oxygen-carrying capacity gives them a training advantage, allowing longer and more intense workouts. Further, at the time of competition, the elevated RBC levels will remain for a few weeks, giving a competitive advantage. Therefore, any bodybuilder who lives at higher elevation and trains in a gym in a valley, will have an advantage.

BLOOD BUFFERING

As most athletes are aware, muscular strength and endurance, decline with time. Depending on the exercise involved, such declines can take seconds, or hours, to occur. Biochemists have a number of theories to account for such declines. The most prevalent theory is that the chief breakdown product of respiration – lactic acid – accumulates, shifting the pH of the blood toward the acid range. This in turn interferes with the muscle's excitation-contraction abilities. Before we go any further, we need to give a brief background in acid/base chemistry.

Living at a higher elevation may give you an advantage. – Michal Klimo

BIOCHEMISTRY 101

Having numerous meanings in day to day living, in chemistry acids and bases have precise definitions. Within solutions there exists varying amounts of negatively charged hydroxide (OH-) ions, and positively charged hydrogen (H+) ions. To compare the proportion of each in a solution, chemists came up with the pH scale. The scale ranges from one to 14, with seven as the neutral point. Those solutions with more H+ ions are placed below seven and are called acid solutions. Those with more OH- ions are placed above seven, and are called basic solutions. The strongest acids rank close to a one, while the strongest bases rank close to 14.

HUMAN APPLICATIONS

Human systems have evolved to work most efficiently at the slightly basic level – between 7.4 and 7.7 on the pH scale. Although it doesn't sound significant, a change of even one small percentage point can have drastic effects on human biochemistry. During exercise, lactic acid buildup, from fatiguing muscles, drags the pH towards the acid side of the scale. And as mentioned earlier, this buildup, and subsequent pH change, is believed to be the main reason for muscular fatigue.

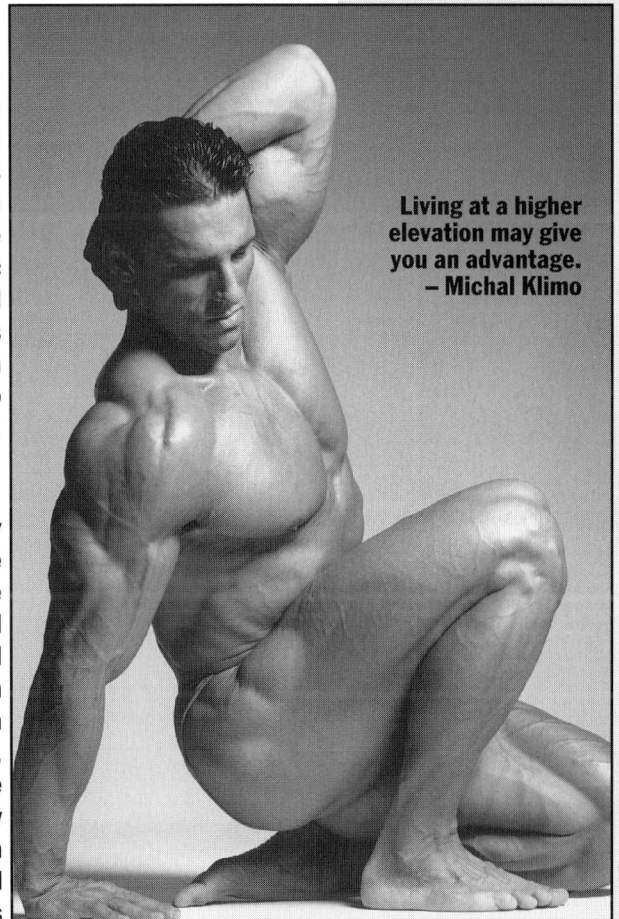

THE BASIS TO A SOLUTION

One of the ways chemists maintain the pH of a solution is by the use of buffers. Buffers are substances that mop up excess ions, thus keeping the pH of a given solution stable. One of the areas of research in athletics is looking for substances that combats the detrimental effects of lactic acid buildup. The one that receives the most attention is called sodium bicarbonate; and while not conclusive, the limited evidence available suggests it can play a role in prolonging muscular fatigue.

Sodium bicarbonate ($NaHCO_3$) works by neutralizing excess H+ ions as they are produced during muscular respiration. If the name sodium bicarbonate frightens you, it's the main ingredient in good old baking soda.

A recent study published in *The Journal of Applied Physiology*, looked at giving sodium bicarbonate in a dosage of 400 milligrams per kilogram of bodyweight to six cyclists. It was found that the test group was able to maintain stronger contractions for longer periods of time than the control non-using group. Further, the experimental group recovered from the exercise quicker than the control group.[3]

We should admit that few studies involving weightlifters have been carried out with sodium bicarbonate. Still given the relative inexpense and availability of sodium bicarbonate, bodybuilders may want to give it a try. Don't expect anything dramatic, but it could get you a couple of additional reps at the squat rack.

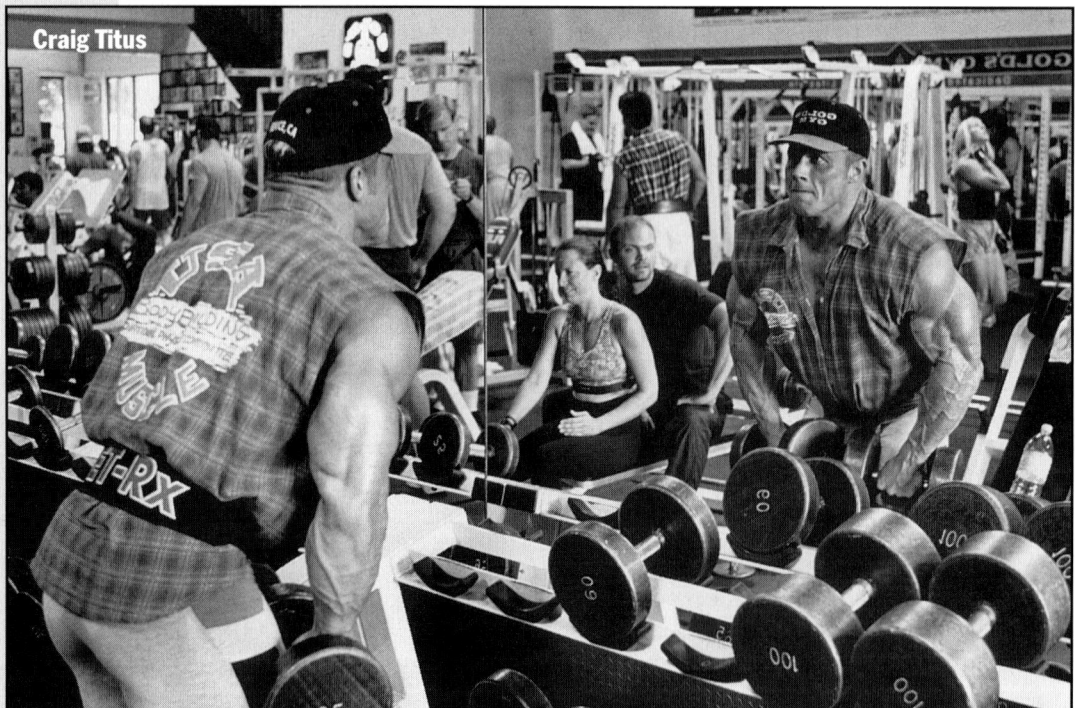

Craig Titus

References
1) Zanca, S. Tour start delayed as cyclists protest. *The Globe and Mail*, p.A26, July 25, 1998
2) EPO, *Drugs, Absolute Truth Hardcore Bodybuilding*, www.geocities.com/Hot Springs/2369/newepo.htm.
3) Verbitsky, O., et al. Effect of ingested sodium bicarbonate on muscle force, fatigue, and recovery. *The Journal of Applied Physiology*, 83 (2) 333-337, 1997.
4) Christie, J. and Freeman, A. Canadian Cyclist watches his dream die, Michael Barry focused his life on winning the Tour de France. *The Globe and Mail, Drugs in Sport, Weekend Edition Sports*, pgs A28 and A25, Nov.7, 1998.

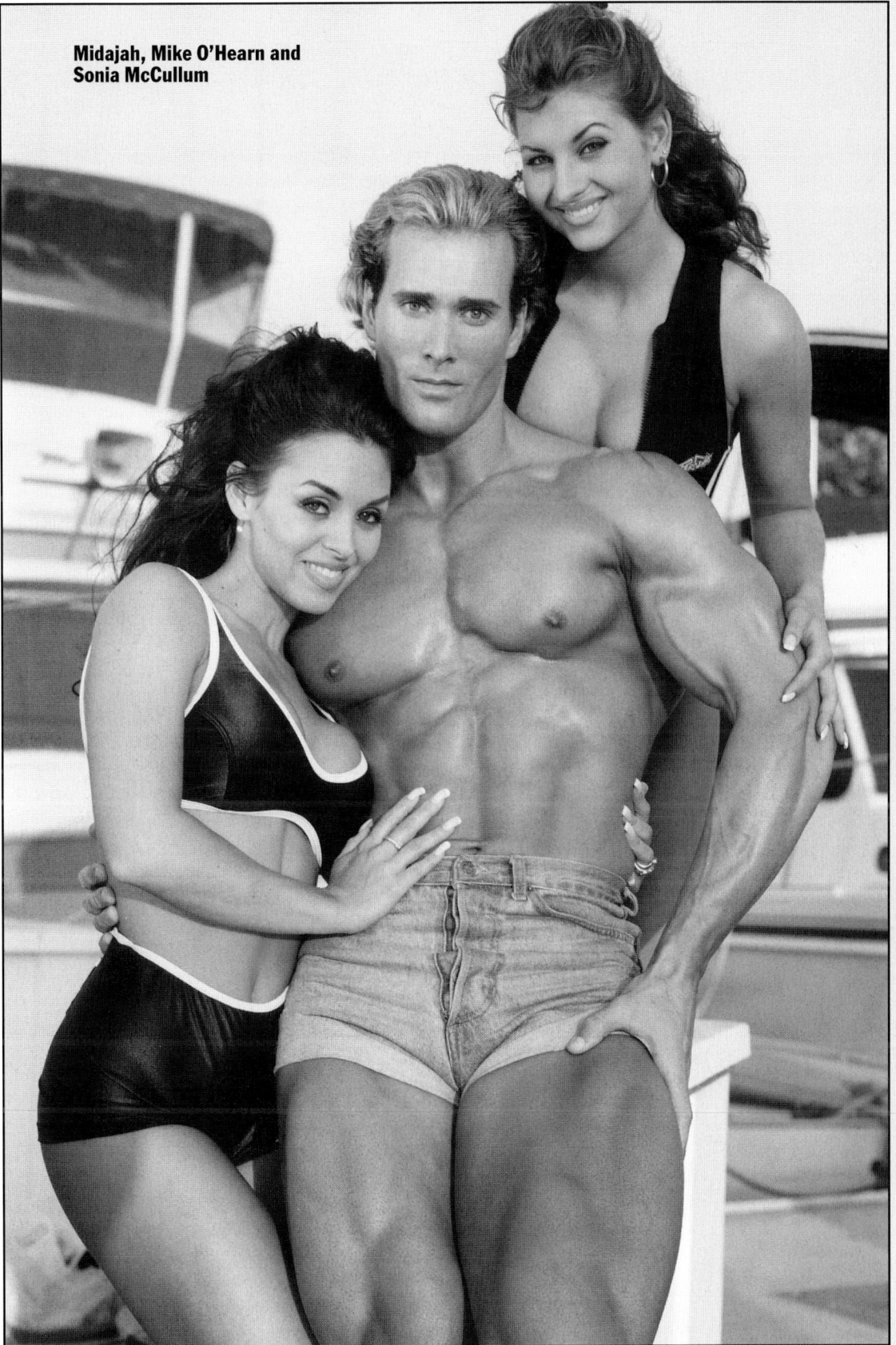

Midajah, Mike O'Hearn and Sonia McCullum

CHAPTER THIRTEEN

Stimulants

We've all had those days where just getting to the gym was a chore in itself, not to mention doing a grueling workout. Most people suffer through such times with a combination of grit and determination. But a few go the extra step and take an over-the-counter stimulant to kick start their system. The drugs of choice are usually ephedrine or caffeine derivatives, but a few brave souls go all the way and try amphetamines.

As the name implies, stimulants are drugs that boost or stimulate the central nervous system or one of its subsystems (i.e. sympathetic nervous system). The end result is increased heart rate, respiratory rate and decreased reaction time. Most over-the-counter stimulants come in the form of cold medications, but the more popular ones like caffeine and ephedrine can also be bought in pure form. In the following chapter we will briefly discuss both over-the-counter and prescription stimulants. Those individuals with heart problems, or a history of heart problems in their family should avoid such drugs. At the very least discuss it with your physician first.

OVER-THE-COUNTER STIMULANTS

This group of stimulants are mainly sympathomimetic amines (nitrogen based), which include ephedrine and its derivatives (pseudoephedrine, phenylpropanolamine and norpseudoephedrine). These drugs are often present as decongestants in cold, hay fever, diet and headache medications – and all are available without a prescription. They work by increasing blood flow and mental stimulation. Adverse effects include elevated blood pressure, headache, increased and irregular heartbeat, anxiety and tremor. Here are some examples:

Amine: Pseudoephedrine
Over-the-counter medications: Actifed, Ambenyl-D, Anamine, Afrin Tablets, Afrinol, Co-Tylenol, Deconamine, Dimacol, Emprazil-A, Fedahist, Fedrazil, Histalet, Isolclor, Lo Tussin, Nasalspan, Novafed, Nucofed, Poly-Histine, Pseudo-Bid, Pseudo-Hist, Rhinosym, Ryna, Sudafed (Very popular with NHL players before a game), Triprolidine, Tussend, Chlorafed, Chlor-Trimeton-DC, Disphoral, Drixoral, Polarmine Expectorant and Rondec

Amine: Phenylpropanolamine
Over- the-counter medications: ARM, Allerest, Alka Seltzer Plus, Contac, Dexatrim, Dietac, 4-way Formula 44, Naldecon, Novahistine, Arnex, Sine-Aid, Sine-Off, Sinutab, Triaminic, Triaminicin and Sucrets Cold Decongestant

Amine: Propylhexedrine
Over-the-counter medication: Benzedrex Inhaler

Amine: Ephedrine
Over-the-counter medications: Bronkaid, Collyrium with
Ephedrine, Pazo Suppository, Wyanoids Suppository and
Vatronal Nose Drops

Comments: Ephedrine is by far the most popular stimulant among body-builders. Athletes use it for both fat loss (see beta agonists) and stimulation. Despite the bad press ephedrine has received over the last couple of years, it is the safest and most effective over-the-counter fat loss and stimulant drug available. The standard dosage for stimulation is 25 to 50 milligrams, 30 to 60 minutes before a workout.

Amine: Herbal Ephedrine (Ma Huang)
Over-the-counter medications: Action Caps, Bishop's Tea,
Breathe Easy Herbal, Decongestant Tea, Brigham Tea,
Chi Powder, Energy Rise, Ephedra, Excel, Free Herbal "Energy
Tablets," Joint Fir, Mexican Tea, Miner's Tea, Mormon Tea,
Popotillo, Quick Shot Vitamin B-12, Squaw Tea, Super Charge
and Teamster's Tea[1]

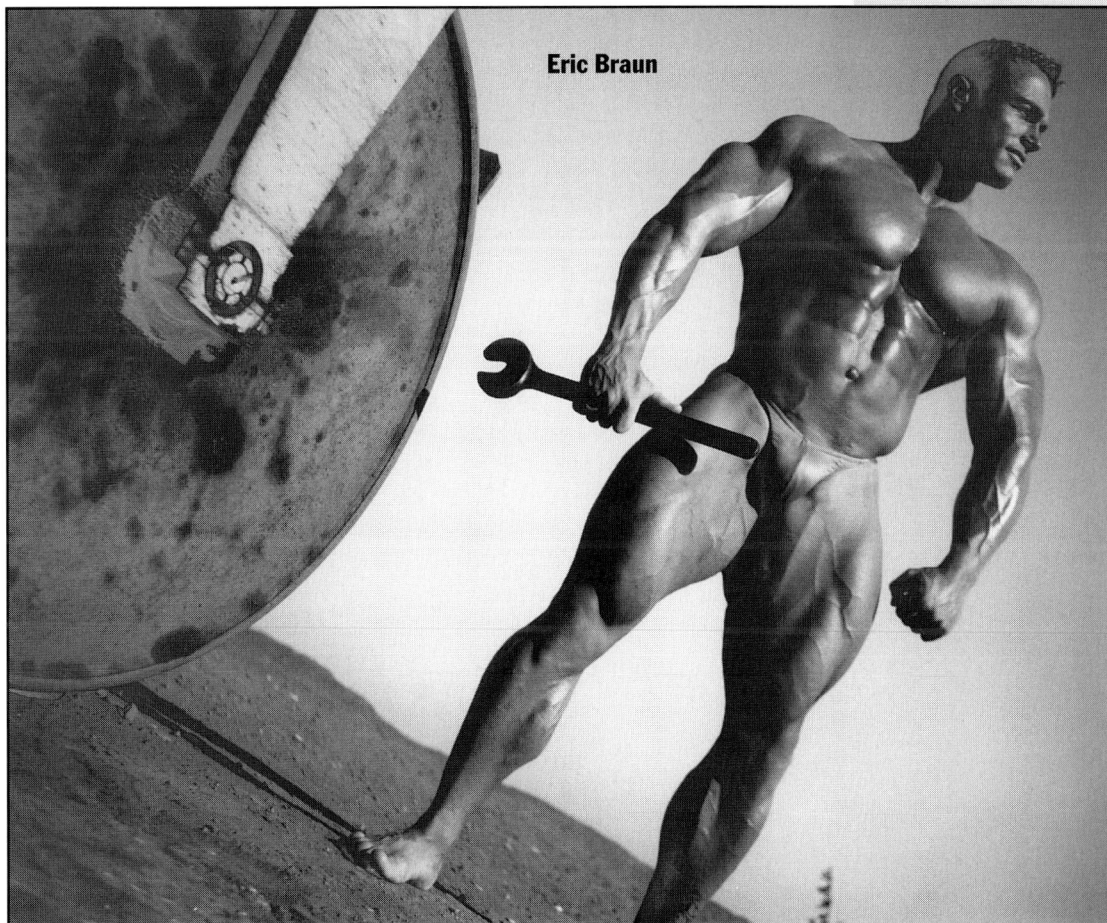

Eric Braun

PRESCRIPTION AMINES

The following are examples of prescription stimulants. They fall into this category for good reason – they are much more powerful than the over-the-counter brands. Of course like just about every drug, they are available on the black market.

Trade Name: Adiposetten N (Germany)
Generic Name: Cathine (Norspeudoephedrine)

Trade Names: Vortel and Asthone (Japan)
Generic Name: Clorprenaline

Trade name: Vicks Inhaler
Generic Name: Desoxyephedrine

Trade Names: Tedral, Bronkotabs, Rynatuss and Primatene
Generic Name: Ephedrine

Trade Names: Mercodal, Decapryn and Nethaprin
Generic Name: Etafedrine

Trade Names: Emivan and Vandid
Generic Name: Ethamivan

Trade Name: Orthoxicol Cough Syrup
Generic Name: Methoxyphenamine

Trade Names: Tzbraine and Methep (Germany and the United Kingdom)
Generic Name: Methyl-ephedrine

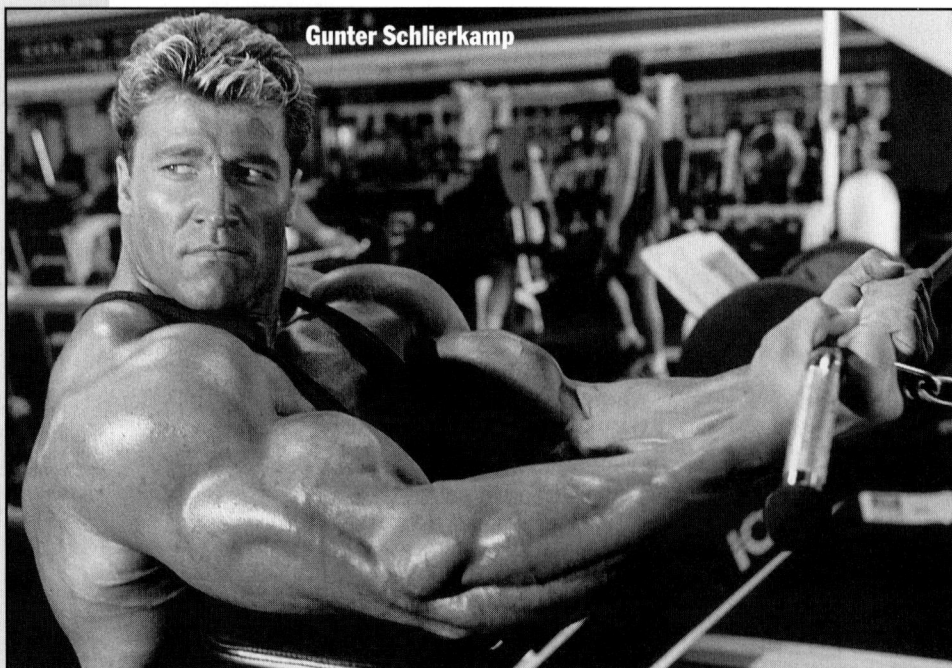

Gunter Schlierkamp

AMPHETAMINES AND RELATED COMPOUNDS

Amphetamines are among the most powerful stimulants. While of limited value to bodybuilders, their use is reported to be rampant in football.

Amphetamines work by increasing alertness, reducing fatigue and possibly increasing competitiveness and hostility. Be aware that some deaths have resulted (even with low doses) under conditions of maximum physical activity. We strongly advise you stay away from amphetamines.

Trade Names: Apistate, Tenuate and Tepanil
Generic Name: Amfepramone

Trade Name: AN-1 (Germany)
Generic name: Amfetamil

Trade Name: Survector (Europe)
Generic Name: Amineptine

Trade Names: Dapti, Daptizole and Amphisol
Generic Name: Amiphenazole

Trade Names: Delcobese, Obetrol and Benzedrine
Generic Name: Amphetamine

Trade Name: Megimide
Generic Name: Bemigride

Trade Name: Didrex
Generic Name: Benzphetamine

Trade Name: Bromantin
Generic Name: Bromantin

Trade Names: Pre Sate and Lucofen
Generic Name: Chlorphentermine

Trade Name: Dinentel (France)
Generic Name: Clobenzorex

Trade Name: Methyl-Benzoylecgonine
Generic Name: Cocaine

Trade Names: Tenuate and Tepanil
Generic Name: Diethylpropion HCL

Generic Name: Cropropamide
Component of: Micoren

Generic Name: Crothetamide
Component of: Micoren

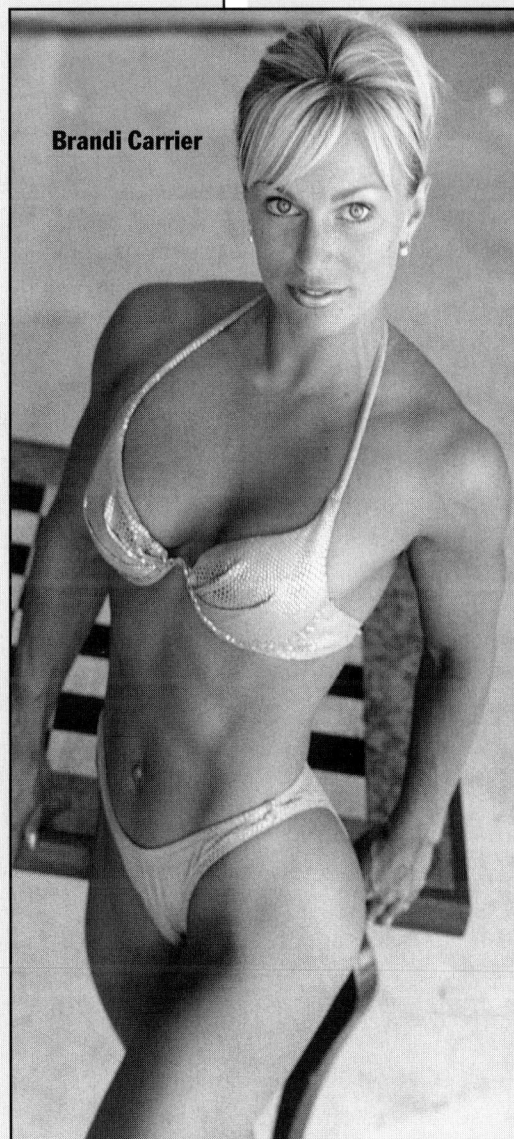

Brandi Carrier

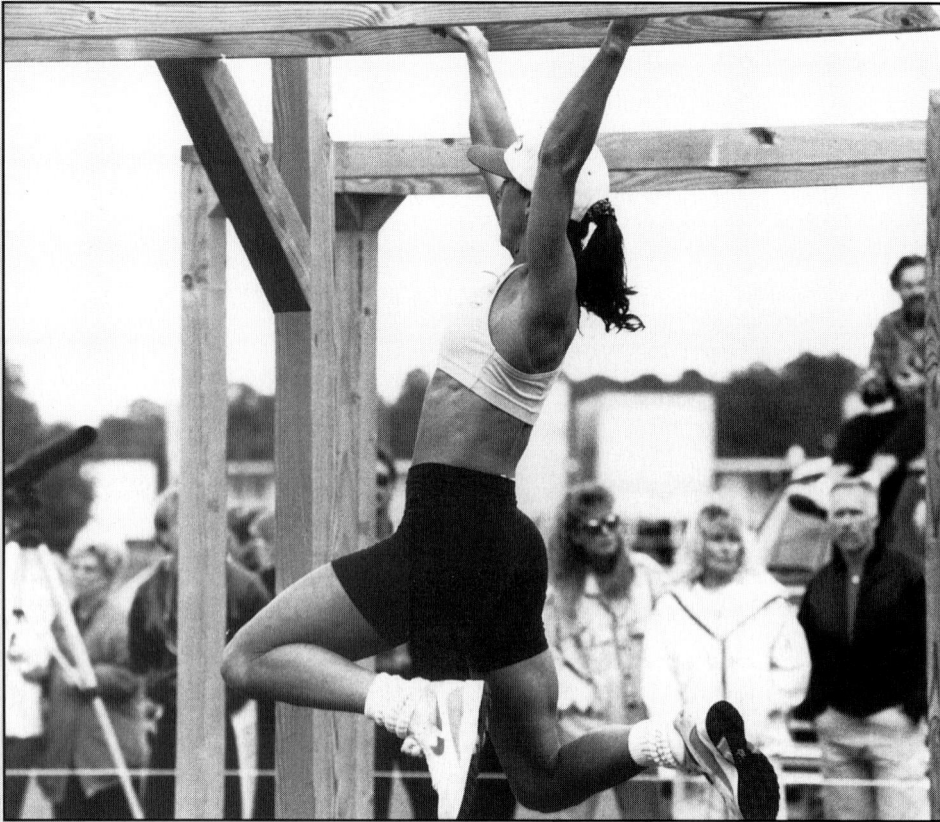

Trade Name: Amphetamine
Generic Name: Dimetamfetamine

Trade Name: Apetinil (Netherlands)
Generic Name: Etilamfetamine

Trade Names: Envitrol, Altimine and Phencamine
Generic Name: Fencamfamine

Trade Name: Captagon (Germany)
Generic Name: Fenetylline

Trade Names: Antiobes Retard (Spain) and
Appetizugler (Germany)
Generic Name: Fenproporex

Trade Names: Frugal (Argentina) and Frugalan (Spain)
Generic Name: Furfenorex

Trade Names: Lucidril and Brenal
Generic Name: Meclofenoxate

Trade Names: Doracil (Argentina), Pondinil (Switzerland)
and Rondimen (Germany)
Generic Name: Mefenorex

Trade Names: Mesocarb, Mesocarbi and Sydnocarb (Europe)
Generic Name: Mesocarbe

Trade Names: Desoxyn and Met-Amphi
Generic Name: Metamphetamine

Trade Name: Rosimon-Neu (Germany)
Generic Name: Morazone

Trade Name: Coramine
Generic Name: Nikethamide (CNS)

Trade Names: Cylert, Deltamine and Stimul
Generic Name: Pemoline

Trade Name: Leptazol
Generic Names: Pentetrazol,
Pentylenetetrazol

Trade Names: Phenzine, Bontril
and Plegine
Generic Name: Phendimetrazine

Trade Name: Preludin
Generic Name: Phenmetrazine

Trade Names: Apidex-P, Fastin
and Ionamin
Generic Name: Phentermine HCL

Trade Name: Cocculin
Generic Name: Picrotoxine

Trade Names: Meratran
and Constituent of Alertonic
Generic Name: Pipradol

Trade Names: Villescon,
Promotil and Katovit
Generic Name: Prolintane

Trade Names: Centroton
and Thymergix
Generic Name: Pyrovalerone

Trade Name: Eldepryl, Plurimen
(Spain) and Deprenyl
Generic Name: Selegiline

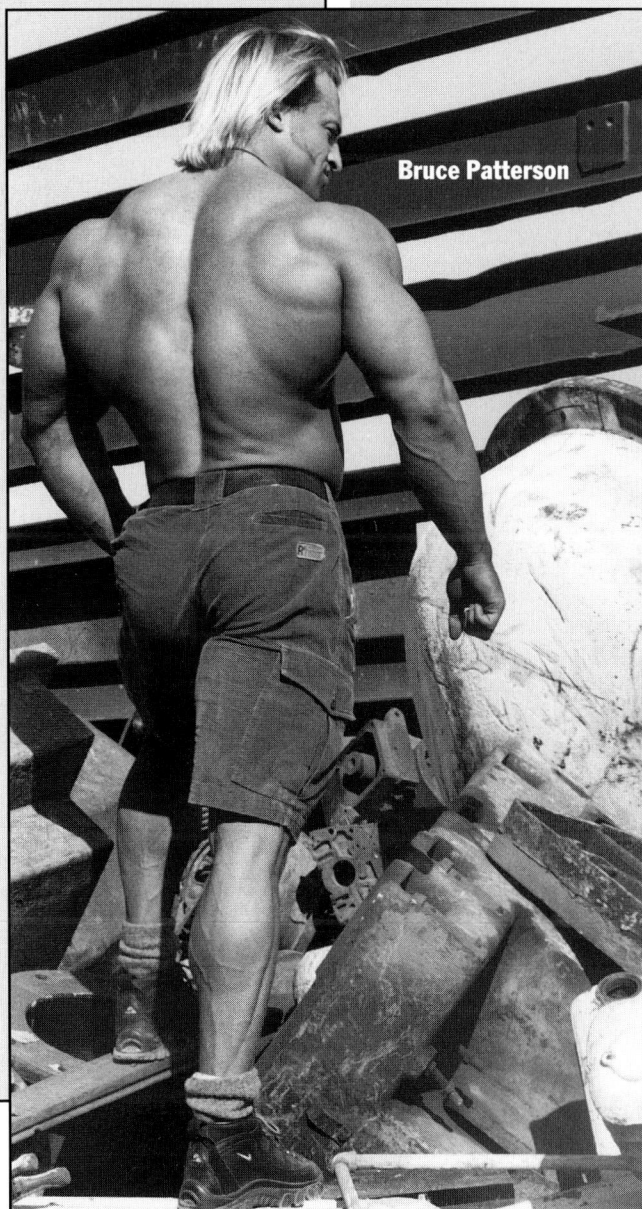

Bruce Patterson

Reference:
1) United States Olympic Committee, Stimulants,
   Drug Control Education,
   http://www.olympic-usa.org/inside/in_1_3_7_1.html.

CHAPTER FOURTEEN

Insulin and Related Drugs

Insulin is a perfect example of just how far some bodybuilders will go for that extra pound of muscle. And the fact that, as of this writing, it is very hard to detect in a drug test hasn't hurt its popularity either.[14] Unfortunately, the drug is also one of the most dangerous and given the wrong set of circumstances could put you in a coma or in a coffin.

WHAT IT IS

Insulin is a peptide (protein) hormone secreted by the pancreas. When blood sugar (and other substances as we shall later see) rise, the brain sends a signal to the pancreas to release insulin. When insulin levels reach a certain point, the brain signals the pancreas to slow down production. Things are not as cut and dry as all this, but for our purposes this is essentially what happens.

> **"Be not the first by whom the new are tried, nor yet the last to lay the old aside."**
> – Alexander Pope.

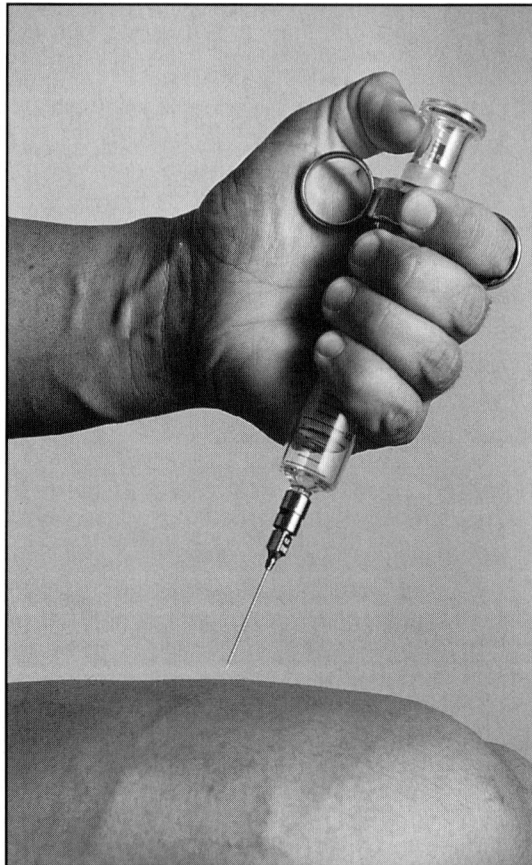

A LESSOR KNOWN FUNCTION

Most readers are probably aware of insulin's role in sugar regulation. Chances are they know someone who has the well-known condition diabetes. Up until the 1920s a diagnosis of diabetes meant almost certain death. Thanks to the works of two Canadian researchers, Banting and Best, the condition is now treatable. Notice we said treatable, not curable. Those with diabetes need to take insulin on a regular basis (determined by the severity of the condition). Still, most diabetics can lead relatively normal lives, provided they watch their sugar intake.

The reason insulin has been added to the bodybuilder's arsenal is because of its role as an anabolic agent! Yes, you read right. Insulin is one of the body's most powerful anabolic hormones. You see insulin does more than regulate sugar, it also speeds the removal of amino acids from the blood stream. More amino acids means more protein synthesis and, there-fore, more muscle building. In a manner of speaking, insulin can be considered a storage hormone.

SOUNDS GREAT BUT...

Now that we've got your attention let's do our best to talk you out of ever trying insulin for the purpose of bodybuilding. Unlike creatine, glutamine or even steroids (despite what the antisteroid groups say), insulin can end your life literally within minutes. Your brain, in addition to your muscles, depends on carbohydrates for energy. Even if you are taking insulin for protein synthesis, it's not a selective hormone. It will still drop blood sugar levels, no matter what you're original intentions. Things may be fine if your sugar levels are high to begin with, but you have no way of knowing. Sure you can pick up a blood testing kit (made for diabetics), but

**The risks of insulin far outweigh the benefits.
– Jay Cutler**

blood sugar is not a static entity. Levels are continuously changing. If blood sugar happens to be low when you administer your insulin shot, you run the risk of dropping it so low you end up in a diabetic coma. If this happens one of three things will occur. If you're lucky, you may come out of it no problem. On the other hand you may survive, but the temporary sugar depletion may have caused brain damage. Finally, the body may never recover and you die. Yes this sounds cold, but you will be cold if you fool around with insulin. We don't think the risk of brain damage or death is a fair trade for a few extra striations or pounds of muscle. And don't think Sammy steroid over in the corner is a fountain of knowledge either. Follow such advice and you could be doing squats at the great squat rack in the sky.

EXAMPLES OF INSULIN DRUGS AND DERRIVITIVES

The following information is for reading purposes only. We strongly advise readers to avoid insulin and related drugs. The risks far outweigh the benefits.

NO MORE NEEDLES – JUST TAKE A DEEP BREATH!

No one likes needles. They're awkward, and they hurt. And then you've got to dispose of them properly. But what if you could just inhale all the insulin you need? It can be done.

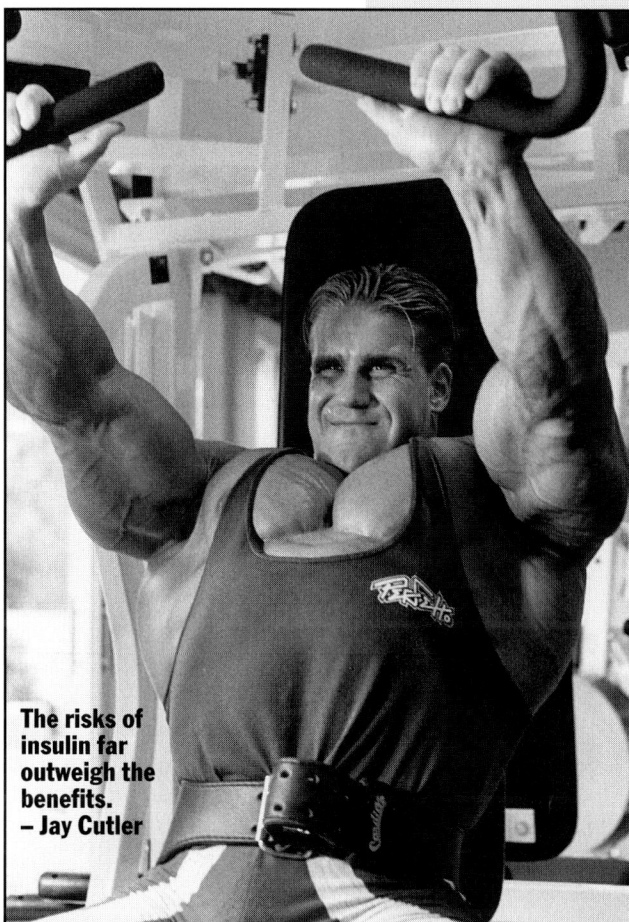

Aerosolized insulin generated by a jet nebulizer delivery system was inhaled continuously by subjects for four minutes. Once in the lungs, insulin rapidly crosses the lung lining into the blood stream. Studies show that pulmonary delivery of inhaled insulin can effectively lower plasma glucose levels.[8] It's still in the early development stages, but in the next few years don't be surprised to see small, insulin inhalers coming on to the market.

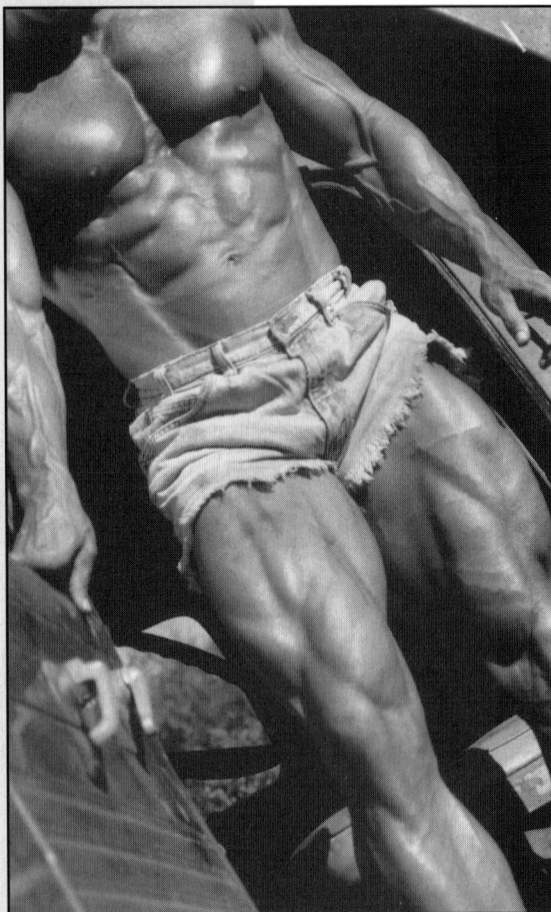

PRAMLINTIDE

Amylin is a peptide hormone that is secreted along with insulin from pancreatic beta cells in response to the ingestion of nutrients. Amylin appears to act on gastric emptying, and to regulate the uptake and use of glucose from food. Even though it has therapeutic promises, human amylin has not been used. It is relatively insoluble, and can aggregate and adhere to various surfaces upon contact. Therefore, amylin derivatives are now being investigated for use in hormone therapy. One currently in use is pramlintide (tripro-amylin or AC137). Selected amino acids are replaced by proline (another amino acid). When administered subcutaneously, pramlintide has been shown to reduce hyperglycemia.[3]

INSULIN LISPRO

This insulin analogue differs from human insulin in that the natural sequence of the amino acids lysine and proline have been reversed. Both lispro and human insulin exist as complex molecules, but following injection, lispro dissociates into simpler molecules more rapidly than human insulin. This facilitates lispro's rapid absorption at the injection site, making it more suitable for mealtime glucose control than regular insulin; since lispro can be administered just before a meal.[10]

RELATED DRUGS AND SUPPLEMENTS

BIGUANIDES

These drugs are antihyperglycemic; which means they make blood sugar levels drop, increasing appetite. Many bodybuilders on anabolic steroids complain of iron stomach; which means that they stop feeling hungry. Biguanides could be a solution to this problem. They work by increasing the transport of blood sugar across the cell membrane into muscle cells. They also increase cellular-insulin sensitivity.[1]

Trade Names: Fenformin, Debeone
Generic Name: Phenformin
Gym Dosage: 150 mg/day, 3 doses of 50 mg, each with water before a meal

Comments: Five to 10 times stronger than Metformin, Phenformin use has declined since it was found to cause lactic acidosis. This disease has a mortality rate of 50 to 75 percent. Same properties as Metformin, except Phenformin also improves pumps and vascularity. Phenformin is very dangerous, thus most bodybuilders prefer to use Metformin.[2]

> Trade Names: Glucophage, Mellitron
> Generic Name: Metformin, Metformin Hydrochloride
> Gym Dosage: 1,700 mg/day in divided doses
> with meals and water, to avoid stomach upset[2]

Comments: Metformin is the most gentle, and least likely of the group to cause Lactic Acidosis (symptoms include: severe cramps, stomach pains and heavy sweating), a potentially fatal condition. This drug can produce the following side effects: nausea, vomiting and metallic taste in the mouth. Metformin enhances the effect of insulin, which itself is an anabolic agent. As it is light and heat sensitive it must be kept refrigerated in a dark place. It takes about six hours to be fully absorbed, and has a half-life of 15 hours. It is safer than oral insulin.

> Generic Name: Insulin-Like Growth Factor I

Comments: IGF-1 seems to have had its day, and is now fading from popularity. There are a number of reasons for this. The first is cost. Genuine IGF-1 is expensive to obtain and reports circulate of pro bodybuilders spending thousands of dollars a month for the stuff. Such cost puts it out of the reach of most athletes. Another reason is effectiveness. On its own IGF-1 doesn't seem to do all that much. It seems to be a good plateau buster when stacked with other drugs like steroids and growth hormone, but on its own it performs poorly. As an example, in one study IGF-I alone failed to reverse protein catabolism. But when IGF-I was combined with HGH (human growth hormone) there was a pronounced anticatabolic effect. Further, this anabolic effect was observed without adverse effects on glucose levels.[11]

> Trade Name: Precose
> Generic Name: Acarbose

Comments: Precose has 100,000 times the binding affinity of glucose for the enzyme alpha-glucosidase. It binds to the enzyme competitively in the small intestine. This enzyme inhibitor exerts its antihyperglycemic activity by slowing the digestion of starches (large complex sugar molecules) into smaller molecules in the upper GI tract, through the inhibition of the enzymes responsible for this conversion.[7,9]

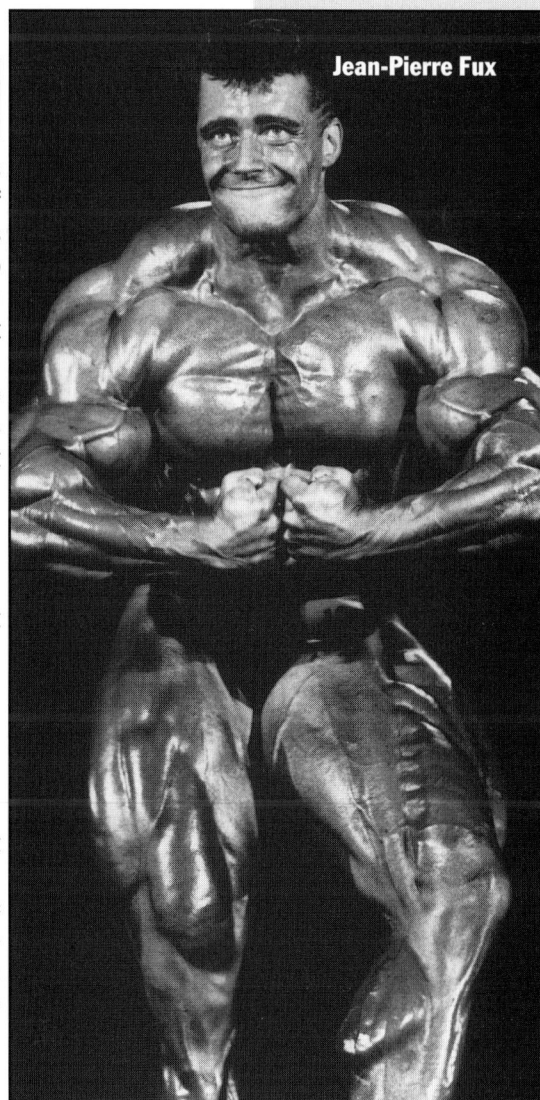
Jean-Pierre Fux

Trade Name: Amaryl
Generic Name: Glimepiride
Dosage: Orally, once daily

Comments: This drug binds to a different site than the other drugs in its class. Amaryl use may result in less elevation of insulin levels over time. It increases both insulin sensitivity and glucose uptake by muscles. It is the only drug in this class that can be taken with insulin.[7]

Trade Name: Prandin
Generic Name: Repaglinide
Dosage: 0.25 mg 3 times daily, taken before meals

Comments: Prandin belongs to a new class of drugs called insulin secreting agents. This drug causes a rapid and short-lived release of insulin by the body. This means that the user can now match his/her own natural insulin release to meal intake.[5]

Trade Name: Rezulin
Generic Name: Troglitazone
Dosage: 200 mg to 600 mg/day, with concurrent reductions in insulin administration

Comments: This drug works by combating reduced insulin sensitivity. It acts at insulin's two major target organ sites, the liver and skeletal muscle. Rezulin appears to affect fatty acid metabolism by targeting receptors called proliferator activated receptors. Glitazone alters the metabolism of fatty acids so that they will not compete with glucose for metabolism. Hence Rezulin lowers blood sugar levels by improving the target cell's response to insulin. The result is a decrease in both glucose production and circulating insulin levels.[6,7] Note: There have been problems reported concerning liver toxicity, so this drug requires close monitoring.

> **"Chromium increases muscle-cell sensitivity to insulin. When muscle becomes more sensitive, the body produces less insulin so carbs can be directed toward the muscles, resulting in decreased fat storage."**
>
> – Greg Zulak, *MuscleMag International* columnist commenting on the role of the popular bodybuilding supplement chromium.

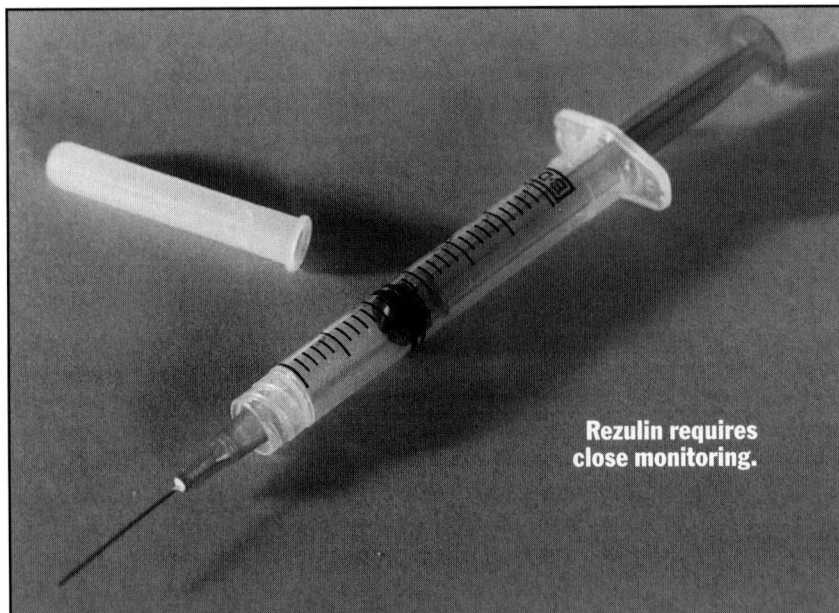

Rezulin requires close monitoring.

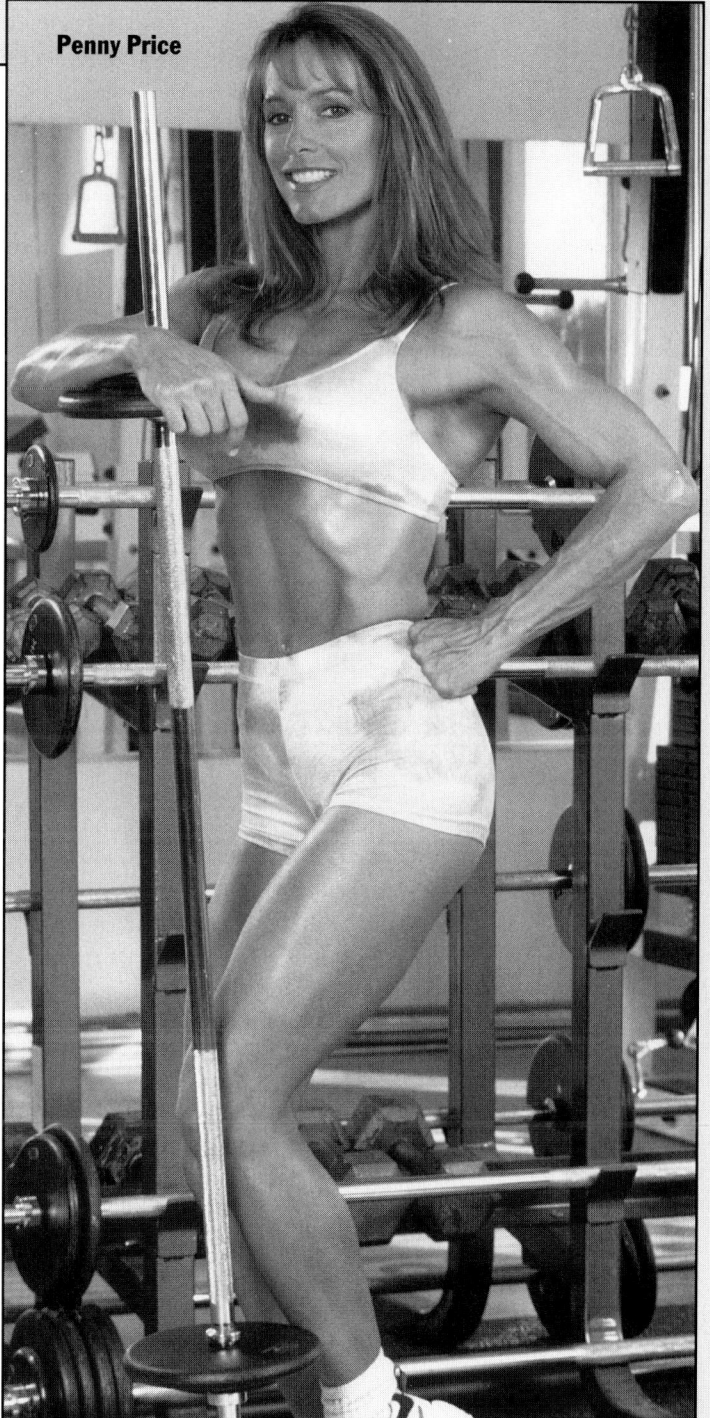

> Trade Name: Meridia
> Generic Name: Sibutramine

Comments: This drug blocks the reuptake of serotonin and norepinephrine. In one study, 50 percent of patients lost 10 percent of their bodyweight after one year. Meridia also causes a decrease in total glucose level.[4]

> Trade Name: Xenical
> Generic Name: Orlistat

Comments: This pancreatic lipase inhibitor causes a 35 percent inhibition of fat absorption, and is correlated with a slight decrease in LDL cholesterol levels. Following a low-calorie diet, users lost 10 percent of bodyweight, and gained back less weight when the diet was no longer restricted.[4]

CHROMIUM

Familiar to most as the shinny metal on expensive sports cars, chromium is also needed by the body for numerous reactions. In bodybuilding circles, chromium gets promoted as an insulin mimicker. From a biochemical viewpoint, this is not entirely true as the element doesn't mimic insulin, but instead assists the hormone in its various regulating roles.

Chromium is believed to work by acting as a coenzyme that somehow boosts the effectiveness of insulin. Studies have shown that individuals deficient in chromium are at risk for decreased muscle metabolism and glucose imbalances.

Exactly how chromium does this is unclear, but recent research in the *Nutrition Review Journal*, helps shed some light on the process. It has been found that complexes with four chromium molecules stimulate enzymes that help bind phosphate groups to proteins. Researchers also found that chromium makes insulin receptors more sensitive to the circulating hormone.[12]

Penny Price

BODYBUILDING APPLICATIONS

Bodybuilders use chromium for two main purposes. As an insulin booster, chromium helps the hormone shuttle nutrients in and out of the blood stream. One such substance is creatine, and there's a volume of anecdotal evidence that chromium speeds creatine absorption. Users report that chromium supplementing gives the muscles a fuller feeling after creatine loading. They also report that the muscles pump up quicker and fuller when using chromium.

The second reason for chromium supplementing is for fat loss. Unlike the previous, which is based on personal interpretation, there is good medical evidence to suggest that chromium can in fact aid in fat burning.

In a recent issue of *Current Therapeutic Research*, scientists gave volunteers 400 micrograms of chromium, and gave a control group an inert (biologically inactive) placebo pill. After controlling the experiment for most variables, the researchers found the group taking the chromium had lost significantly more fat and bodyweight than the control group. What made the study so relevant was that neither group knew what they were taking.[13]

USING CHROMIUM

As there are no RDA's established for chromium, our recommendations are based on the average amounts used in most medical studies. Generally speaking, you should take 200 to 400 micrograms of chromium per day. As with most supplements, space the dosages out over the day, with numerous smaller dosages.

We should add that chromium can come in a number of different forms; the most popular being chromium picolinate. Other versions include chromium citrate, chromium chloride and chromium polynicotinate. A few magazine articles have raised the issue of picolinate's safety, but the studies cited involved megadosing. The fact that the particular magazine's publisher had their own form of chromium didn't make their argument very convincing. In our opinion there's very little difference between the various forms. One nice thing about chromium supplementing is it's cheap. Twenty bucks will get you over a month's supply.

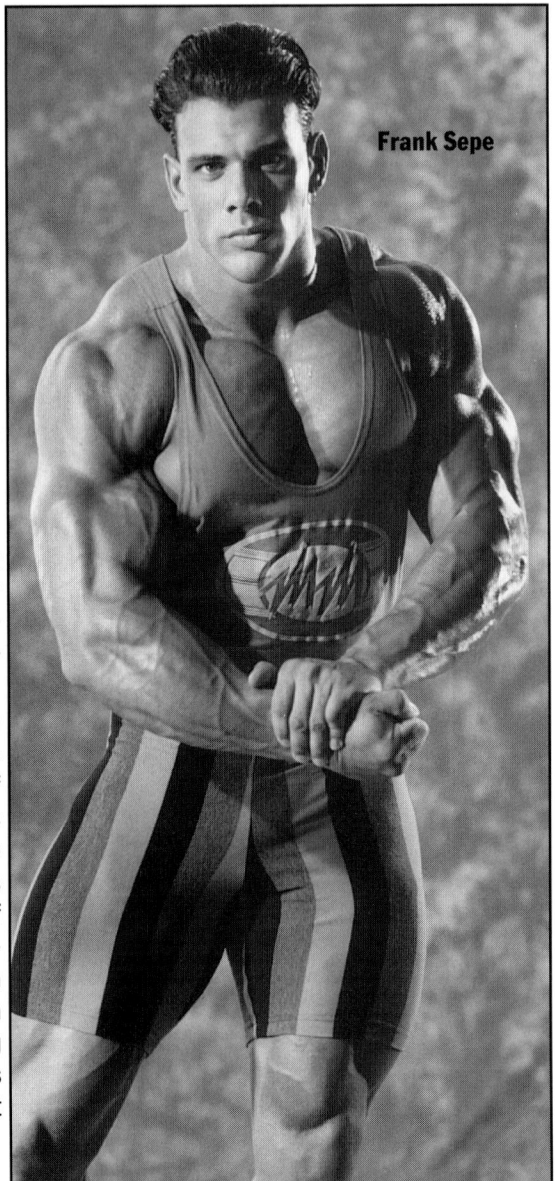

Frank Sepe

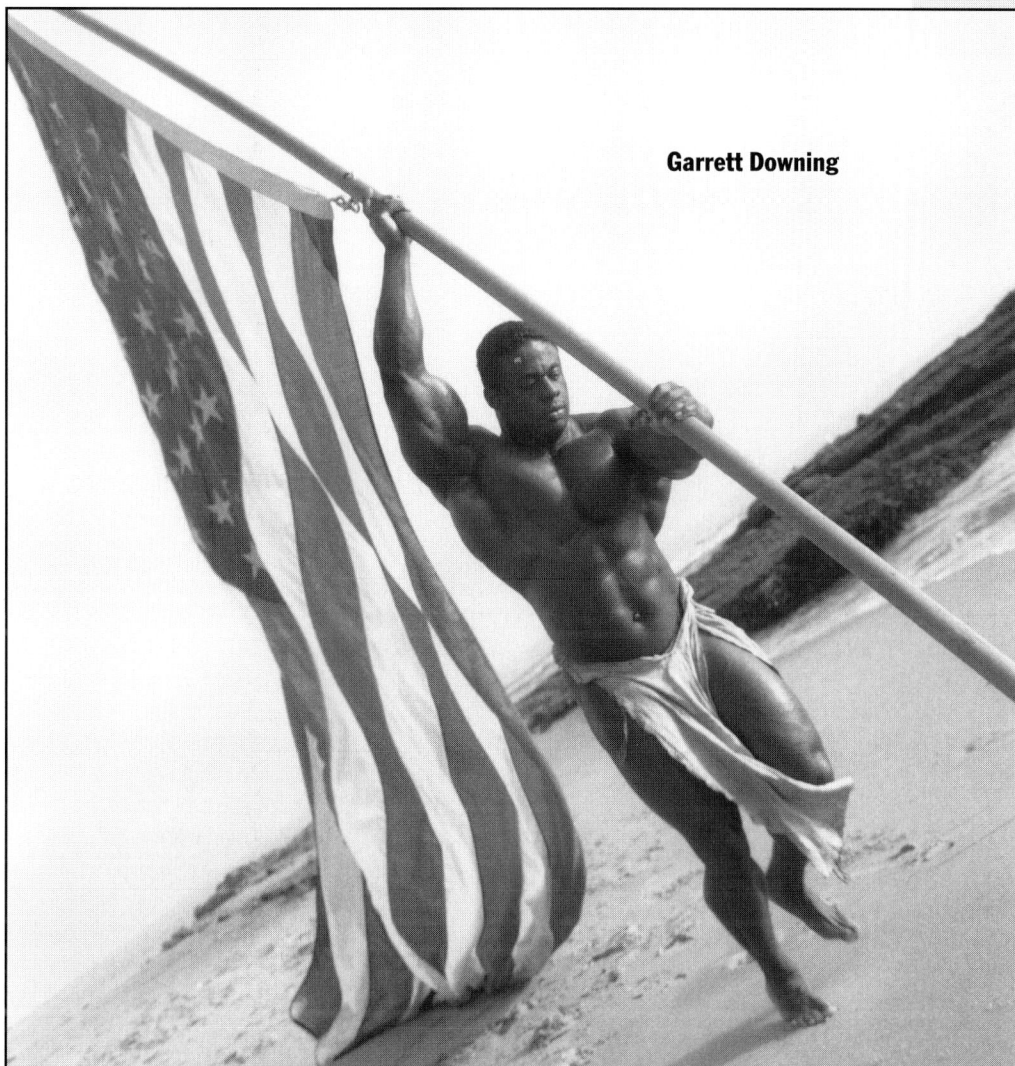

Garrett Downing

References
1) Glucophage, extract from The Big Secret, *Battle News*, Issue 16, http://www.ironpages.com/Glucophage.html.
2) Glucophage, Drugs, *Absolute Truth Hardcore Bodybuilding*, http//www.geocities.com/HotSprings/2369/newglucophage.htm.
3) Thompson, R., Pearson, L., Gottlieb, A., and Kolterman, O. Pramlintide, an Analog of Human Amylin, Can Reduce Fructosamine in Patients with Type I Diabetes, Diabetes 1996 *Electronic Highlights Bulletin* #3, June 10, 1996, http://ARMINFO.COM/disease/diabetes/ehlb/ehb1_3.html#2.
4) Drug Treatment of Overweight Diabetics, http:/PHARMINFO.COM/disease/ADA97/ADA-7103.html.
5) Repaglinide: An Investigational Drug For Diabetes, http://PHARMINFO.COM/disease/diabetes/ADA97/ADA-7113.html.
6) Troglitazone Approved for Control of Hyperglycemia in Type II Diabetes, http://PHARMINFO.COM/pubs/msb/troglit237.html.
7) New Approaches to the Pharmacotherapy of Diabetes, http://PHARMINFO.COM/disease/diabetes/eh1b/ehb1_2html#6.
8) Laube, B. and Benedict, G. Nebulized Inhaled Insulin: A new approach to managing glucose levels, http://PHARMINO.COM/disease/diabetes/eh1b/eh1b_2.html#6 .
9) Committee Recommends Acarbose for NIDDM, http://PHARMOINFO.COM/pubs/msb/acarbose.html.
10) Anderson, J., Brunelle, R., Pfeutzner, A. et al Reducing the Incidence of Hypoglycemia with a Novel Insulin Formulation, http://ARMOINFO.COM/disease/diabetes/chlb/ehb1_1.html#8.
11) Berneis, K., Ninnis, R., Girard J., Frey, B. and Keller, U. Effects of Insulin-Like Growth Factor I Combined with Growth Hormone on Glucocorticoid-Induced Whole-Body Protein Catabolism in Man, *The Journal of Endocrinology & Metabolism*, 82, 2528-2534, 1997.
12) Mertz, W. Interaction of chromium with insulin: A progress report, *Nutrition Review*, 1998, 56: 174-177.
13) Kaats, G.R., Blum, D., et al. A randomized, double-masked, placebo-controlled study of the effects of chromium picolinate supplementation on body composition: A replication and extension of a previous study, *Current Therapeutic Research*, 1998, 59, 379-388.
14) *The Lancet*, June 21, 1997, 349.

CHAPTER FIFTEEN

Thyroid Drugs

Darin Lannaghan

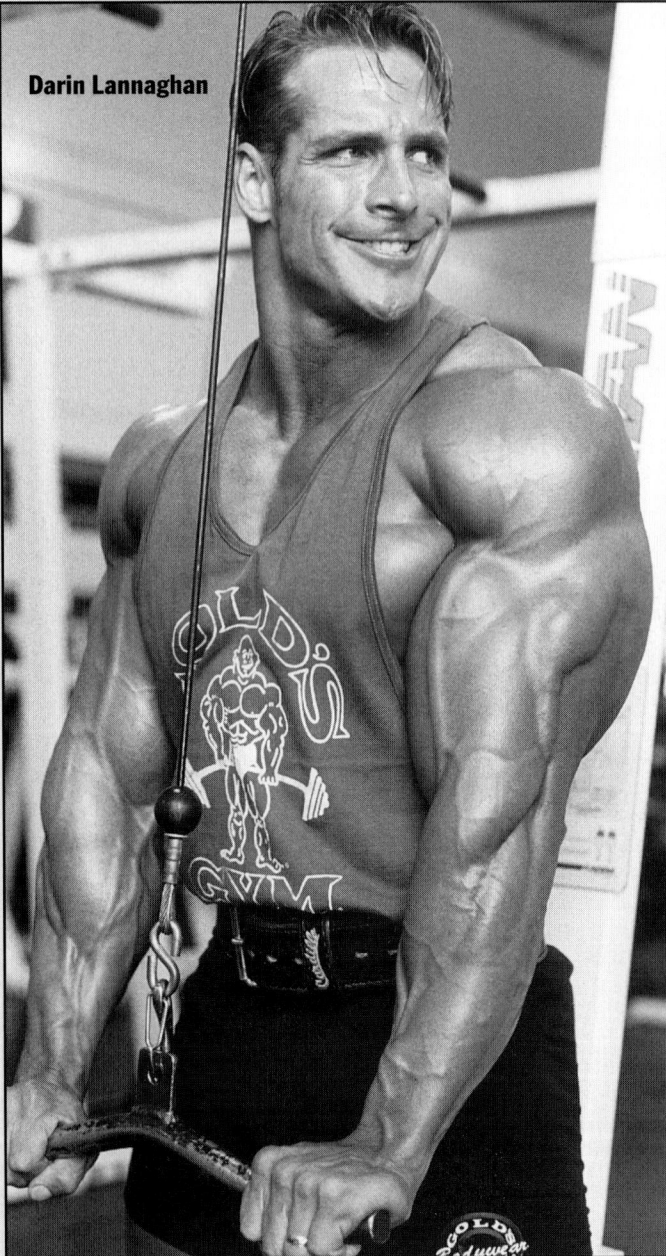

Flip through a recent copy of *MuscleMag International* and compare the photos of today's bodybuilders with their counterparts of 20 or 30 years ago. Not only are today's stars bigger, but their miniscule level of bodyfat makes their physiques look like something out of *Gray's Anatomy*. It's not uncommon for today's bodybuilders to step on stage sporting bodyfat down in the two to three percent range. Does this mean today's bodybuilders know more about diet and cardio than competitors did 20 years ago? Probably not. The difference is in available pharmacology. And at the forefront of fat fighting are thyroid drugs.

WHAT THEY ARE

It has long been known that there's a relationship between obesity and thyroid irregularity. The thyroid gland is a small organ located in the neck, to the front and side of the trachea (windpipe). The thyroid gland is primarily made up of two types of cells. The most prevalent are the follicular cells, which secrete two thyroid hormones: tri-iodothyronine (T3) and thyroxine (T4). The other types of cells, called parafollicular, secrete calcitonin, a hormone responsible for calcium regulation. For the purposes of this book, we'll limit our discussion to T3 and T4.

Although T4 accounts for about 90 percent of thyroid output, T3 is more concentrated and, therefore, just as effective. Both hormones are primarily composed of the amino acid tyrosine and the common element iodine. Although there's slight differences, both hormones seem to contribute to the same functions. These can be generalized as follows:

• Acceleration of cellular reactions.
• Increase in body metabolism.
• Increase in the cardiovascular system.
• A role in mineral and water regulation.

Of the previous the one that gets the most attention from bodybuilders is the second, the overall increase in body metabolism. Thyroid hormones increase the rate at which the body uses oxygen for cellular reactions, thus raising the body's temperature and giving off heat and energy. When things work properly (and calorie intake and energy expenditure are kept constant) the thyroid gland does an excellent job of keeping bodyfat levels fairly constant. It's when things malfunction that the fun starts. How often have you heard an overweight individual say they've got a glandular problem? Now in the majority of cases, the problem is a lack of exercise and poor eating habits. But occasionally there is a problem with the thyroid. For our purposes, the end result of such a malfunction is slowing the body's metabolic rate, and the consequent gaining of many pounds of bodyfat (in some cases hundreds of pounds – check out the *Guinness Book of World Records* – over a thousand pounds in a couple of cases). Of course the opposite is also true, and an overactive thyroid will burn bodyfat like crazy. Are you now beginning to see why bodybuilders are interested in thyroid drugs?

Since thyroid drugs are readily available for those suffering thyroid disorders, bodybuilders usually have no problem obtaining them on the black market. All it takes is a few tablets to go from a normal metabolism to a fat burning machine. It's easy to see now why bodybuilders these days are turning up on stage looking like medical charts. Of course, as expected, there is a downside.

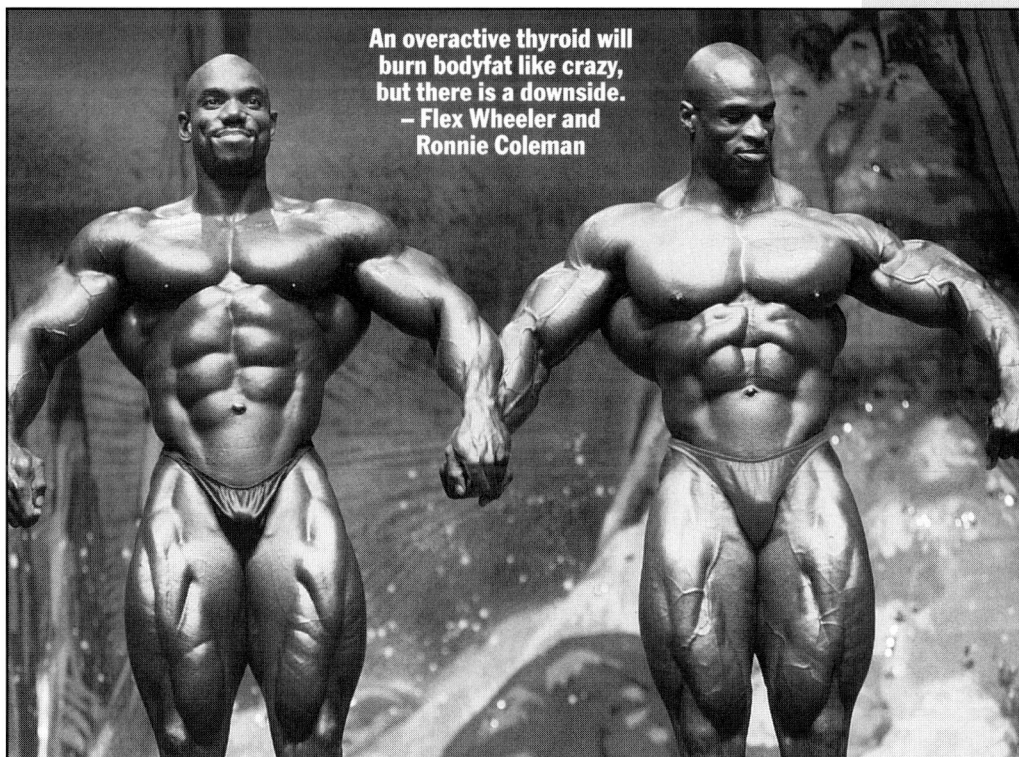

An overactive thyroid will burn bodyfat like crazy, but there is a downside. – Flex Wheeler and Ronnie Coleman

THE BOOMERANG EFFECT

Like most of the body's hormones, the thyroid hormones are controlled by a process called biofeedback. Basically the body monitors its own levels of circulating thyroid hormones. As soon as levels drop, the brain tells the thyroid to increase production. When levels reach a certain height, the brain tells the thyroid to slow down. In effect there is a delicate balance between too much and not enough. As soon as you introduce a foreign variable into the equation (in this case extra thyroid) this delicate balance is thrown off.

Numerous stories are told of former bodybuilders and fitness contestants who are now life dependent on thyroid drugs. Basically their use of thyroid drugs damaged their own system's ability to manufacturer T3 and T4. They found this out the hard way after coming off the drugs. Within weeks they put on dozens of pounds of bodyfat. Even months later their own systems still had not cut in and an examination determined that the damage was such that they would need to use thyroid for life. Once again the question becomes, is it worth screwing up your hormonal system just for the loss of a few extra pounds of bodyfat?

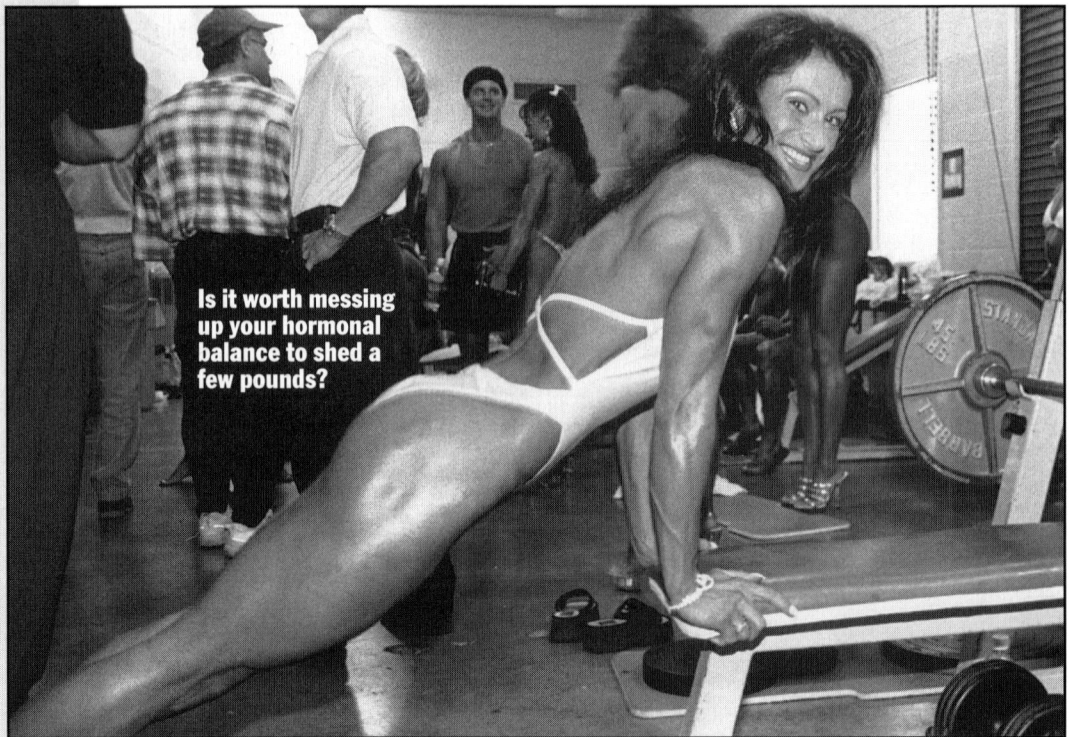

Is it worth messing up your hormonal balance to shed a few pounds?

USING THYROID MEDICATION

Despite our recommendations not to, we know there are readers who will experiment with thyroid drugs. The following is not meant to be taken as gospel but used as a rough guide.

Trade Names: Cynomel, Cyronine, Cytomel, Cytomel Tabs, Euthroid, Lincomel, Liothyronin, Neo-Tiroimade, Ro-Thyronine, Tertroxin, Thybon-Forte, Thyrotardin, Ti-Tre, Tiromel, Tironina, Trijodthyronin, Trijod.Sanabo, Trijodthyr.50, and Trijodthyr.L

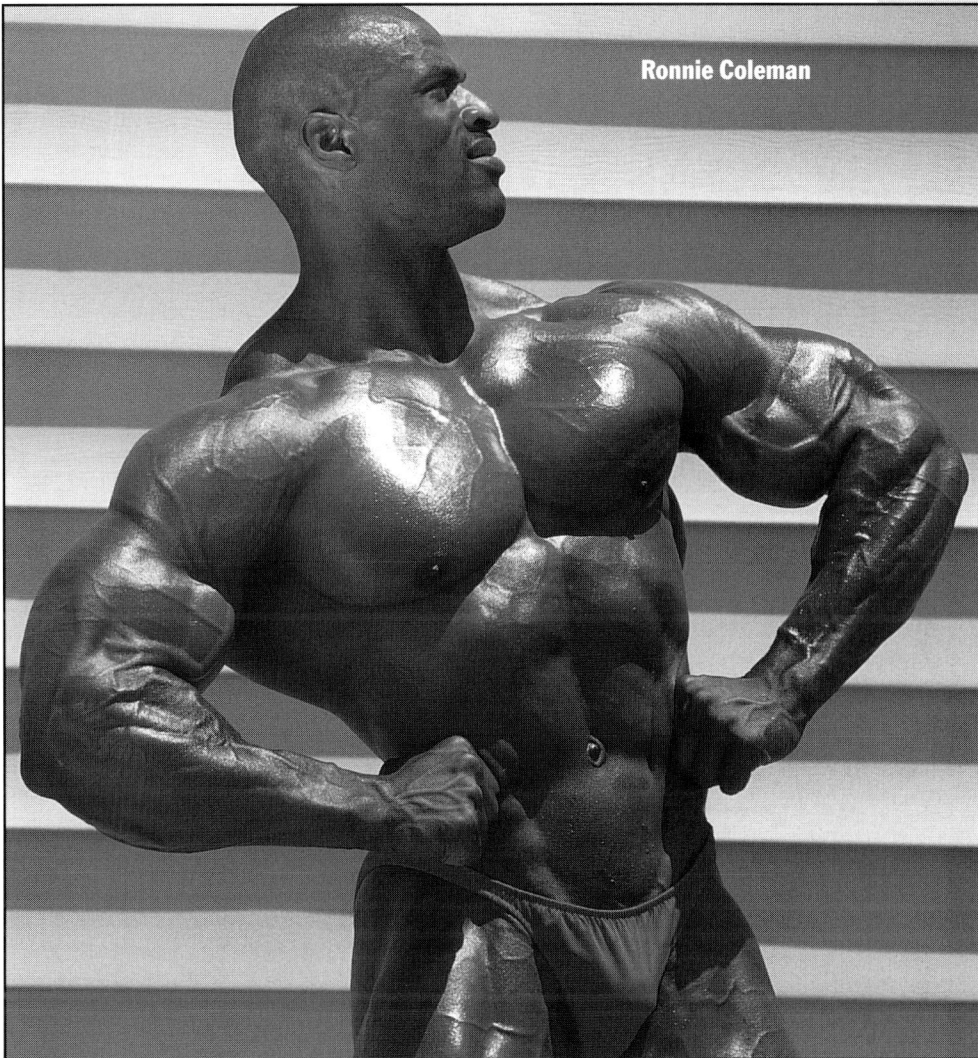

Ronnie Coleman

Day One – 37.5 micrograms of T3, 50 micrograms of T4 and 20 milligrams of ephedrine.

T3 and T4 have a half-life of three days, so to prevent system shut-down, stay with a one day on / one day off cycle. Insulin can be added to this stack, but caution is advised. Thyroid hormones have a hypoglycemic effect, therefore, sugar levels must be monitored and your diet adjusted accordingly.[1]

An alternative method is to start at 25 micrograms per day of T3, increasing by 25 micrograms per day, every five to six days. Do not exceed 100 micrograms per day. Make sure to take T3 in evenly divided doses throughout the day (100 micrograms would be divided into four doses of 25 micrograms). The user must cycle down when going off this drug to maintain normal thyroid function. This drug should not be taken longer than five weeks, and one should wait at least eight weeks before using T3 again.[2]

References:
1) Uncovering the Metabolism Myth, *Battle News, Issue 16,* http://www.ironpages.com.
2) Cytomel, *Absolute Truth Hardcore Bodybuilding,*
   http://www.geocities.com/HotSprings/2369/newcytomel.htm.

CHAPTER SIXTEEN

Nutrient Update

The following can be considered a hodgepodge of the latest information pertaining to common food nutrients. We are not going to go into detailed biochemistry on each nutrient group, such information can be found in *Anabolic Primer*. Instead we'll briefly mention some of the latest research studies, and the implications for bodybuilders and other athletes.

MAGNESIUM

Magnesium is like zinc, copper and chromium, in that the body only needs it in small amounts. But it plays a pivotal role in numerous metabolic reactions, in particular both nerve conduction and muscular contraction. In patients with magnesium deficiency there is a marked reduction in these systems. And the latest research published in the *Journal of American College Nutrition*, has found that athletes may also be at risk.

Twenty-six marathon runners were tested for magnesium after completing a long distance run. They were found to have significantly lower magnesium levels than the control groups. Researchers suggest that intense exercise causes increased magnesium uptake by the muscles, which in turn left less available for other systems.[1]

With regards to dosage, the accepted amount is 500 to 1000 milligrams per day. Unlike the debate over chromium forms, all forms of magnesium are absorbed easily by the body, so don't be too concerned by brand names.

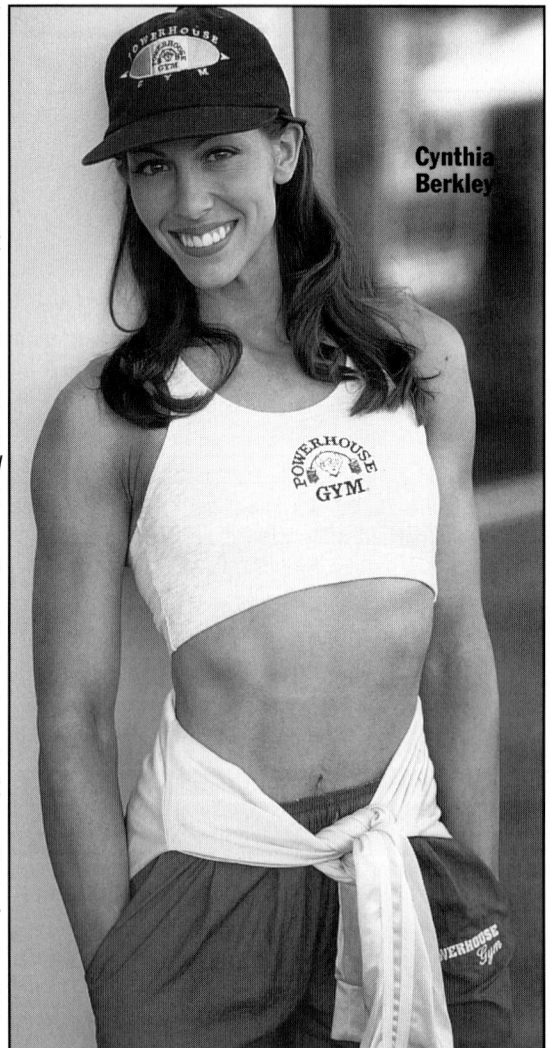

Cynthia Berkley

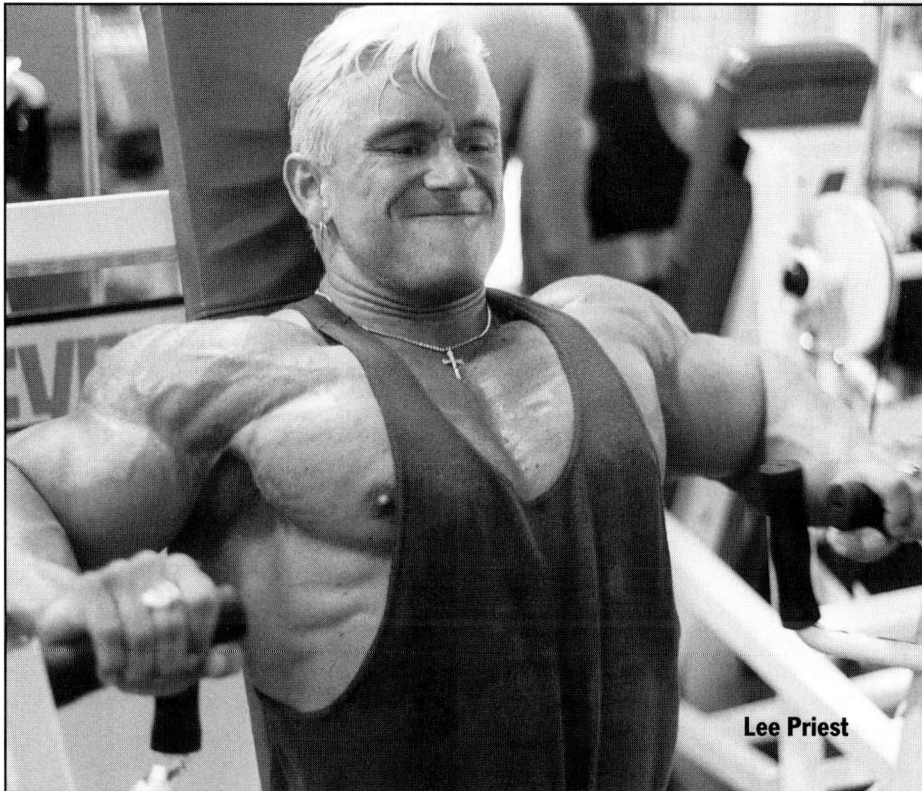

Lee Priest

CARBOHYDRATE – FORM AND STATE

One of the big debates in athletics these days is whether high or low glycemic index carbs are best for providing energy. As a quick review, high glycemic index (high GI) carbs are absorbed very quickly, while low glycemic index (low GI) carbs take longer. A recent study in *Medicine and Science in Sports and Exercise* has helped shed some light on this topic.

Two groups of cyclists were given a high or low GI carb supplement before a 50-minute cycling program. The researchers found no difference between the two groups with regard to cycling performance.[2]

We should add that because high GI carbs cause a more rapid insulin release, and consequently a reduced level of lipolysis (the use of fat as a fuel source), those trying to lose weight should stick with low GI carbs before working out (at least for exercise lasting under an hour).

Besides type, the state of carb supplements (i.e. solid versus liquid) has come under suspicion. In other words does a liquid sport's drink like Gatorade offer a quicker source of energy than a carbohydrate sport's bar? A recent study published in *Sport's Medicine Digest* offers a surprising opinion.

The researchers gave two groups of athletes either a liquid carbohydrate drink or a solid sports energizer bar. It was assumed that the liquid group would perform better on tests, but the researchers were surprised to find that both groups performed equally well. Further, blood sugar and insulin levels were also equivalent. The conclusion is that liquid sport's drinks do not offer athletes an advantage when it comes to supplying a quick source of energy.[3] The only possible drawback to sport's bars is that some athletes find food makes them nauseous during physical activity.

"I found it hard to keep a straight face and say nice things about soy, as I had always considered it basically a waste of time for bodybuilders."

– Will Brink, regular *MuscleMag International* writer and author commenting on his interview with a Japanese film crew about the benefits of soy protein.

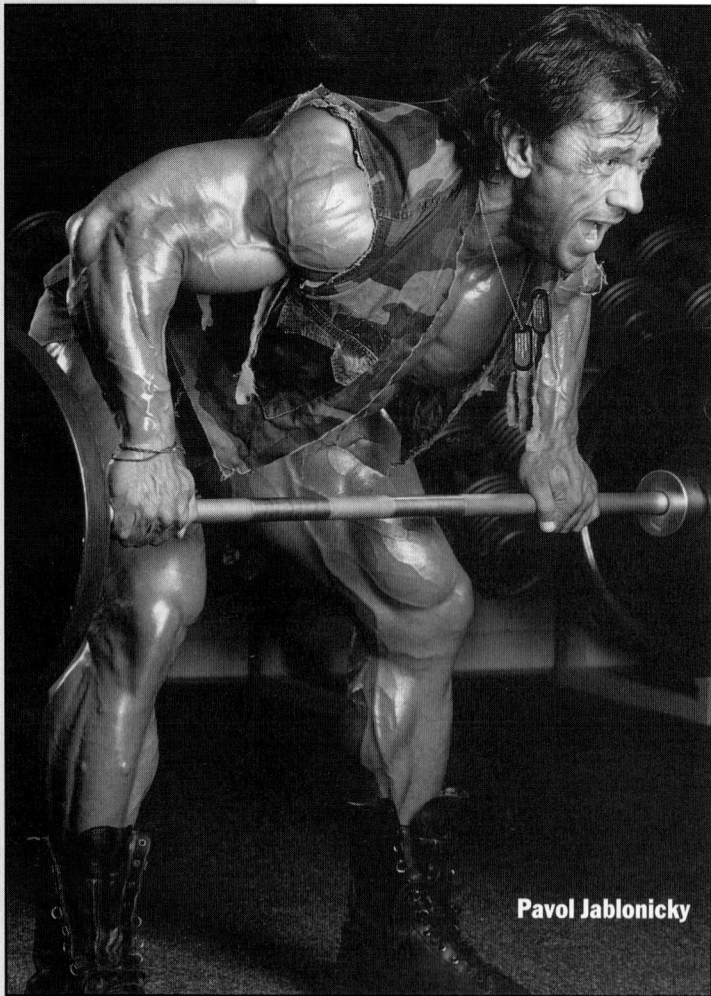

Pavol Jablonicky

THE GREAT SOY PROTEIN COMEBACK

It's funny how some things come full circle. When we finished writing *Anabolic Primer* over two years ago, soy protein had but all been dismissed by the supplement industry. Yet two years later this lowly plant protein is making a fast comeback.

The fall of soy protein started with the introduction of milk and egg protein sources in the 1960s and 70s. Animal sources are superior because they offer the full compliment of amino acids, whereas plant sources are usually missing one or more of the aminos. This is why vegetarians must consume a wide range of plant sources to get the full compliment of amino acids in their diet.

Before the redemption of soy, we should touch on the main reasons why it was dismissed for so many years. The first strike against soy is it scores low on the BV scale – a 74 to be exact. For those not familiar with the scale, it measures the amount of protein deposited as opposed to the amount absorbed. To quote Will Brink: "High BV proteins are better for nitrogen retention, immunity response, IGF-1 stimulation and are superior for reducing tissue loss during various wasting states."

This last part is important as it basically means high BV proteins keep catabolism to a minimum. In terms of ranking, whey protein ranks highest, followed by whole eggs, followed by soy sources.[4]

Another drawback to soy is it lacks the amino acid methionine. What's one amino acid you say? Well methionine plays a major role in protein synthesis, immune response and the manufacture of glutathione – one of the body's main antioxidants.

A third strike is that soy may block the absorption of many nutrients. One theory is that soy interferes with proteases – the body's main protein for digesting enzymes.

Finally, soy has always been known (at least since research started examining protein sources in detail) to be high in estrogenic compounds – substances that increase bodyfat storage.

BUT WAIT

For those not turned off by soy and still wanting to read more, let us now see if we can bring soy back from the dead, so to speak.

Let's start with the last point, the one about high estrogenic substances. Studies with animals found that such compounds have little or no effect on the animals' reproductive hormones. In short, animals that ate soy had no differences compared to control animals not eating soy. More important, estrogenic compounds are known to lower cholesterol levels (one of the primary reasons why women have less heart disease than men).[5]

Also related to this topic is evidence to suggest that small amounts of estrogen may make testosterone receptors more receptive to the male hormone. The result is an increased anabolic effect from the same amount of testosterone.

The issue of soy interfering with nutrient metabolism has been addressed by supplement manufacturers. Those properties that reduce nutrient absorption and metabolism have been removed during soy refinement and production.

With regards to soy's deficiency in methionine, this has easily been solved by adding it during the manufacturing process – much the same way many breakfast cereals are fortified with vitamins and minerals.

A new area of soy research focuses on the protein's possible cancer fighting properties. A recent study published in the *Journal of the National Cancer Institute* suggests soy contains an anti-cancer compound called genistein. Researchers theorize that genistein blocks the production of proteins that permit cancer cells to grow.[7]

Finally, there is limited evidence to suggest soy protein can, at least in animal studies, raise thyroid hormone levels.[6] Now if human studies start finding the same, soy may help bodybuilders shed fat during the pre-contest season.

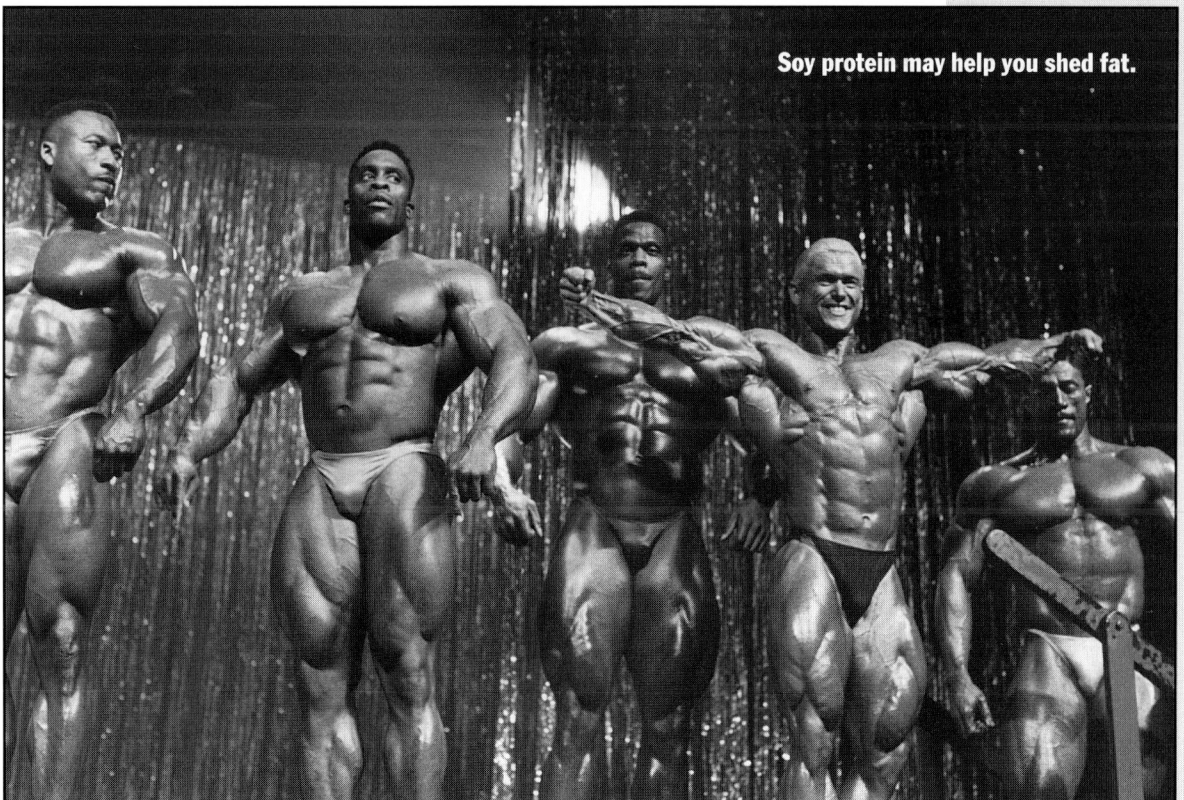

Soy protein may help you shed fat.

INCORPORATING INTO YOUR DIET

The nice thing about supplementing with soy is that you don't seem to need to consume mega doses – say in the 25 to 30 grams per day range. This does not mean, however, you replace egg or whey protein with soy. Take Will Brink's advice and add it to your egg or whey protein shake in a ratio of one part soy to two parts whey or egg. You now get the superior muscle and immunity boosting properties of whey with the cholesterol lowering, thyroid stimulating properties of soy. The perfect protein supplement combination.

WHEY MORE ON WHEY

Whey protein is a perfect example of how far the supplement industry has come over the last few years. Although bantered about for decades it was only in the late 1980s and the early 1990s, that whey protein really took off.

Without repeating what we said in *Anabolic Primer*, suffice to say whey protein is the best protein available. Period. Yes, soy has its advantages and egg proteins have stood the test of time, but whey surpasses all of them in virtually every category.

As would be expected the days of going into a store and only having one form of whey to choose from are over. Whey protein comes in three different forms – based for the most part on manufacturing technique. Hopefully after reading the following you'll be able to choose the one that meets your needs.

WHEY PROTEIN CONCENTRATE

Of the three, whey concentrate is by far the most commonly used in the supplement manufacturing industry. There is a good reason for this and that's cost. Whey concentrate is the cheapest of the three to produce. It is also of a slightly lesser quality as it contains more fats and carbohydrates than the other two. This may explain why some users experience gastric discomfort when taking it. Of course it's still far more digestible than some of the old protein concoctions of years gone by.

For those who track their protein intake to the nearest gram, keep in mind that 30 grams of whey concentrate is about 70 percent actual protein – about 21 grams. The other nine grams are carbs, fats and other by-products. Still of the three, whey concentrate is probably the best value for your dollar, and a few extra carbs and fat is not going to hurt most people.

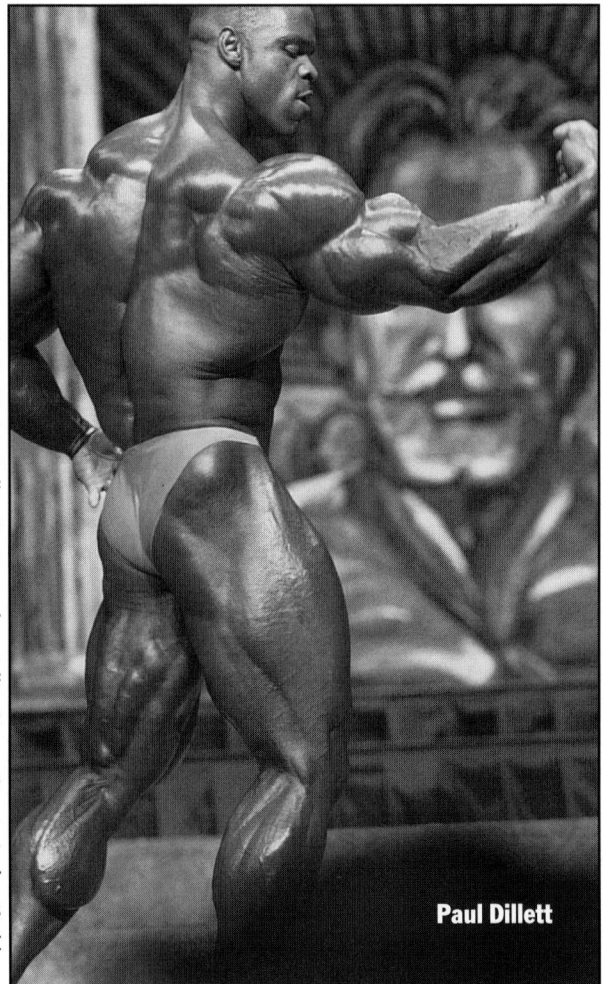

Paul Dillett

WHEY PEPTIDE OR HYDROLYZED WHEY

In terms of absorbability and digestibility, whey peptide is probably the best. This is because, in a manner of speaking, it's partially digested for you. The protein molecules have been broken down (or hydrolyzed) into peptides during the manufacturing process.

If hydrolyzed whey has a disadvantage, it's cost – averaging two to three times more than whey concentrate. It's also very bitter in the pure form unless mixed with some sort of artificial flavor. Still if money is no object, hydrolyzed whey is state of the art.

WHEY ISOLATE

Falling somewhere between concentrate and peptide, are the two whey isolates – ion exchange and microfiltration. Ion exchange is formed by separating the

Whey protein is still the best. – Renita Harris

protein, based on electrical charge. As the various milk proteins are passed through a reaction tank, they are drawn to various resins, depending on their electrical charge. This process produces a protein supplement that is 90 to 95 percent protein by volume. This purity makes whey isolate among the most digestible of wheys, and doesn't usually produce the gastric problems sometimes seen with concentrate forms.

Microfiltration isolate is produced by passing the protein mixture through ceramic filters that remove excess fats, carbohydrates and other unwanteds. The end result is 95 to 98 percent protein by volume. One of the added bonuses of microfiltration wheys is that they're almost totally lactose free. This means those lacking the enzyme to digest lactose (a milk sugar) don't need to take digestive enzymes.

THE RIGHT WHEY

Given the high quality of the three types of whey protein we are not going to recommend one over the other. Even the lowest quality of the three, whey concentrate, is superior to the other popular proteins such as whole milk, egg and soy. We should add the trend these days is for manufacturers to add all three types to their protein supplements.

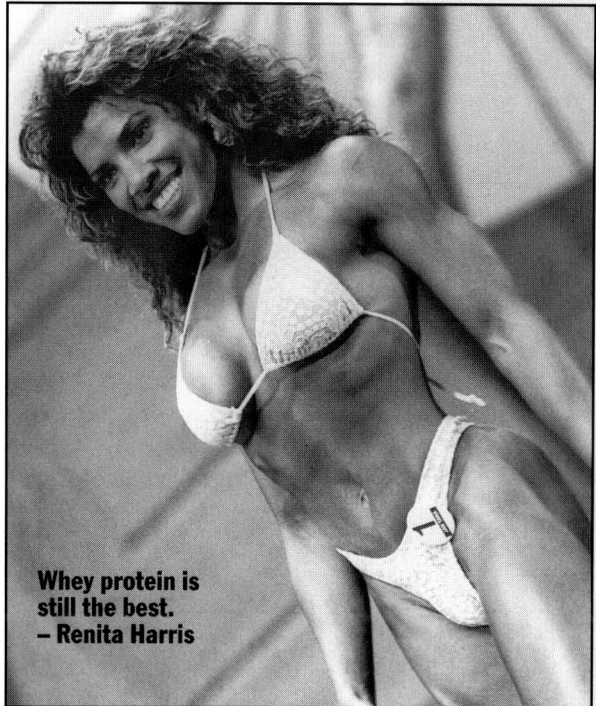

References
1) Buchman, A.L., et al. The effect of a marathon run on plasma and urine mineral and metal concentrations. *Journal of American College Nutrition*, 17: 124-127, 1998.
2) Sparks, M.J., et al. Pre-exercise carbohydrate ingestion effect of the glycemic index on endurance exercise performance, *Medicine and Science in Sports and Exercise*, 30:844-849, 1998.
3) Coleman, E. Liquid versus Solid Carbohydrate feedings, *Sports Medicine Digest*, 20: 68-69, 1998.
4) Brink, Will. The Partial Redemption of Soy Protein, *MuscleMag International*, Aug, 1997.
5) Anthony, A.S., et al. Soybean isoflavones Improve Cardiovascular Risk Factors Without Affecting The Reproductive Systems of Peripubertal Rhesus Monkeys, *Journal of Nutrition*, 125: 43-49, 1995.
6) Forsythe, W.A. Soy Protein, Thyroid Regulation and Cholesterol Metabolism, *Journal of Nutrition*, Supplement 125 (3) 619S - 623S, 1995.
7) Zhou, Y., Lee, A.S. Mechanism for suppression of the mamalian stress response in genistein, an anti-cancer phytoestrogen from soy. *Journal of the National Cancer Institute*, 90, 381-388, 1988.
8) Gang of Five, □www.testosterone.net/QUE/html/gof6.html.

CHAPTER SEVENTEEN

Historical Anabolics

We thought it amusing to end the book with a few short stories illustrating how doping and ergogenesis are not products of the 80s and 90s. Whenever money, power and prestige was at stake, some individuals employed every trick in the book to insure they came out on top. Although common sense should prevail when reading these anecdotes, a few readers may be willing to take things too seriously. As you'll see we advise against such foolhardiness.

"I take the fifth."

– Just about anyone in organized crime, in a U.S. court, who wanted to stay alive.

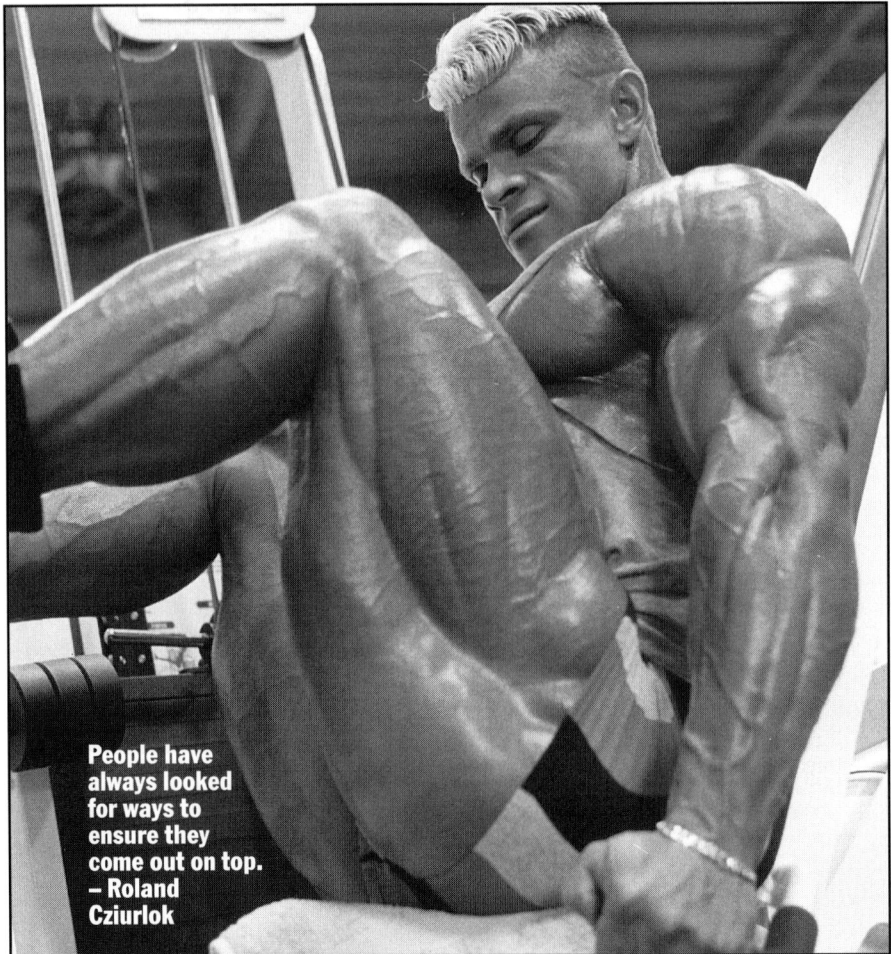

People have always looked for ways to ensure they come out on top. – Roland Cziurlok

HUMAN POWERED HORSES

Classical Greek mythology tells us about Diomedes, son of Aries and Cyrene. His horses were fed a special diet to make them savage and unbeatable. However, we don't recommend this one. If you think laws on anabolic steroids are strict, check out the ones regarding cannibalism. The horses owned by Diomedes ate human flesh.[1]

DID BEN HUR HAVE AN EDGE?

During the time of the Roman Empire, chariot racing was among the most popular of spectator sports (right up there with gladiator fighting and feeding the politically incorrect to the lions). Naturally, this sport attracted gamblers, who were always looking for an edge. A doping mixture called hydromel (honey and water) was given to horses to make them run faster. We don't know how effective it was (perhaps pollen from local flowers contained a stimulant), but Roman officials appear to have been convinced of hydromel's efficacy. The punishment for its use was crucifixion.[1]

DID BIG AL PLACE A BET?

In 1932, horserace betting was legal in only eight states, but later that year legalized betting was permitted in 20 more. The result was a boom in doping. One such prescription survives:

Heroin	1.5 g
Strychnine	2.5 g
Nitrogylcerin	10 minims
Tinct. Digitalis	5 minims
Cola nut	2 oz

One half of this dose was to be given 50 minutes before the race, and the other half 30 minutes later. The heroin would limber up a sore horse, and the caffeine would act as a stimulant.[1] WARNING – this combination would either result in a coma or death in a human, so we don't recommend you try this one.

Bill Davey and Trish Stratus

"What should I do in Rome? I am no good at lying. If a book's bad, I can't praise it, or go around ordering copies.

I don't know the stars; I can't hire out as an assassin when some young man wants his father knocked off for a price. . ."

– Juvenal writes, making observations about life in Rome.

Reference
1) Tobin, T. *Drugs and the Performance Horse*, Charles C.Thomas, Publisher, Springfield, Illinois, 1981.

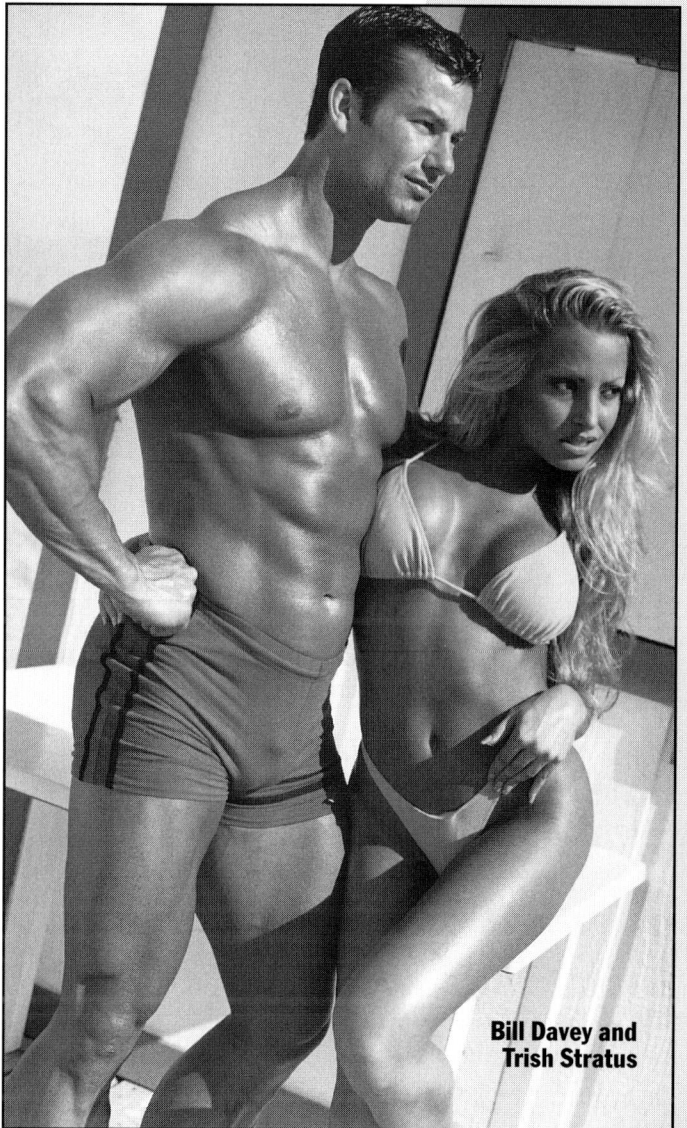

Appendix

TYPICAL DRUG COMBINATIONS FOR BUILDING MASS AND STRENGTH

Dianabol + Primobolan Depot
Gossips have it that this combination could grow muscles
on an Austrian Oak.[4]

Primobolan + Deca-Durabolin + Sustenon 250[4]
Primobolan + Durabolin + Sustenon 250[15]
Primobolan + Laurabolin + Sustenon 250[12]

Synovex-H + testosterone
Synovex-H + Dianabol
Synovex-H + Anadrol 50
Good results.[5]

Finaplix-H + testosterone
Finaplix-H + Dianabol
Finaplix-H + Anadrol 50
Good results.[6]

Equipoise + Anadrol
Equipoise + Dianabol
Equipoise + Sustenon 250[7]

Parabolan + Any Testosterone[10]

Masteron + Metandiabol
Masteron + Reforvit-B
Masteron + Parabolan[11]

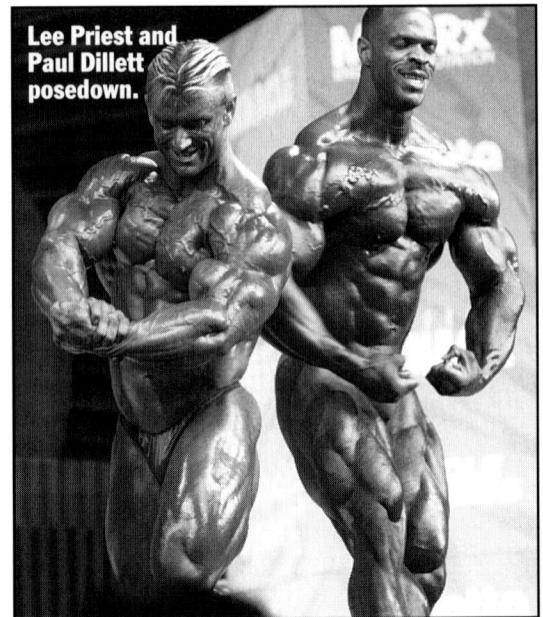

Lee Priest and Paul Dillett posedown.

Primobolan Depot + Sustenon 250 + Laurabolin[12]
Primobolan Depot + Sustenon 250 + deca-durabolin[13]
Primobolan Depot + Sustenon 250 + Durabolin[15]

Dianabol + deca-durabolin[16]
Dianabol + Laurabolin[12]
Dianabol + Durabolin[15]

Anavar + Sustanon 250
Anavar + Testosterone Cypionate[17]

Methandriol + Any Testosterone Injectable
Methandriol + Maxibolin
Methandriol + Metandren[18]

Weeks 1 to 2: Halotestin dns
Weeks 3 to 4: Testosterone Enanthate dns
May result in gynecomastia and permanent
testicular shrinkage.[2]

Weeks (not specified): Sustenon 250 to 500 mg/week,
Dianabol 20mg/day,
Nolvadex dns, Proviron dns
Followed by:
Weeks 1 to 8: Testosterone Enanthate 250 mg/week,
Nolvadex dns, Proviron dns
Weeks 9 to 12: Testosterone Enanthate 250 mg/week,
deca-durabolin
400 mg/week, Nolvadex dns, Proviron dns
Week 13: Testosterone Enanthate 250mg/week, Orimetin dns,
Nolvadex dns, Proviron dns
Weeks 14: HCG 5,000 i.u. three times daily, Clomid dns, Nolvadex dns,
Proviron dns
Weeks 15 to 16: HCG 5,000 i.u five times daily, Clomid dns, Nolvadex dns,
Proviron dns
Weeks 17 to 24: Spiropent dns
Claims to have avoided the steroid crash.[2]

Weeks 1 to 10: Drive 2 ml/week, Dianobol 50, 50 mg/week
User went from 74 to 80 kgs, with a loss of bodyfat.[19]
Anadrol-50 + deca-durabolin[21]

Week 1: 1/2 tab Anadrol-50, 100 mg deca, 20 mg nolvodex
Week 2: 1 tab Anadrol-50, 200 mg deca , 20 mg nolvodex
Week 3: $1^{1}/_{2}$ tab Anadrol-50, 300 mg deca, 10 mg nolvodex
Week 4: 1 tab Anadrol-50, 300 mg deca, 10 mg nolvodex
Week 5: 1/2 tab Anadrol-50, 200 mg deca, 10 mg nolvodex
Week 6: 100 mg deca, 5 mg nolvodex.

Note: The previous is an outstanding size stack. Unfortunately, the Anadrol-50 makes it extremely toxic to the liver as well. And despite the nolvodex, there's a good chance some conversion to estrogen will take place.

Primobolan + Sustanon + D-bol + Proviron[22]
Week 1: 100 mg Primobolan
Week 2: 200 mg Primobolan
Week 3: 200 mg Primobolan, 1 amp sustanon
Week 4: 300 mg Primobolan, 1 amp sustanon
Week 5: 300 mg Primobolan, 2 amp sustanon
Week 6: 300 mg Primobolan, 2 amp sustanon
Week 7: 300 mg Primobolan, 1 amp sustanon, 40 mg d-bol/day,
25 mg proviron/day
Week 8: 200 mg Primobolan, 1 amp sustanon, 30 mg d-bol/day,
25 mg Proviron/day
Week 9: 200 mg Primobolan, 1 amp sustanon, 10 mg d-bol/day,
25 mg Proviron/day

Week 10: 2500 iu HCG, 25 mg Proviron/day
Week 11: 2500 iu HCG, 80 mg clenbuterol/day
Week 12: 120 mg clenbuterol/day

PRE-CONTEST CYCLES

DRUG COMBINATIONS FOR GETTING CUT AND/OR HARD

Primobolan + Winstrol + Testosterone Undecanoate[4]

Parabolan + Anavar[4]
Parabolan + Deca-Durabolan[10]
Parabolan + Durabolin[15]

Synovex-H + Winstrol
Synovex-H + Stromba[5]

Finaplix-H + Winstrol
Finaplix-H + Stromba[6]

Equipoise + Parabolan
Equipoise + Halotestin (NOT RECOMENDED)
Equipoise + Winstrol[7]

Primotestin Depot + Anavar
Primotestin Depot + Primobolan[8]
Provirion + Teslac
Proviron + HCG
Proviron + Clomid
Increases muscle hardness.[9]

Masteron + Winstrol-Depot
Adds hardness and definition to the muscles.[11]

Primobolan Depot + Winstrol + Androil[13]
Cutting cycle.
Winstrol + Sustenon 250
Winstrol + Testosterone Cypionate
Cutting cycle.[14]

Weeks 1 to 5: Cytadren 250 mg/day, Deca 350 mg/week,
Winstrol-V 175 mg/week, Suspension 350 mg/week
Week 6: Cytadren 250 mg/day, Deca 350 mg/week,
Winstrol-V 175 mg/week, Primobolan Depot 300 mg/week
Weeks 7 to 10: Cytadren 500 mg/day, Deca 350 mg/week,
Winstrol-V 175 mg/week, Primobolan Depot 300 mg/week,
Clenbuterol dns
Week 11: Cytadren 250 mg/day, Deca 200 mg/week, Clenbuterol,
Clomid 250 mg/day
Weeks 12 to 13: Cytadren 250 mg/day, Clenbuterol,
Clomid 250 mg/day[1]

Week 1: D-bol (Dianabol, 5 mg/tab), 2 tab/day, T-Cyp (testosterone cypionate, 200 mg/ml) 200mg/week
Week 2: D-bol 3 tab/d, T-Cyp 300 mg/week
Week 3: D-bol 4 tab/d, T-Cyp 400 mg/week
Week 4: D-bol 3 tab/d, T-Cyp 300 mg/week
Week 5: D-bol 2 tab/d, T-Cyp 200 mg/week
Week 6: D-bol 1 tab/day
Week 7: HCG 5,000 i.u.
Week 8: HCG 5,000 i,u.[3]

Deca-durabolan + Dianabol[20]
Week 1: 100 mg injection, 2 tabs/day
Week 2: 200 mg injection, 3 tabs/day
Week 3: 300 mg injection, 4 tabs/day
Week 4: 400 mg injection, 5 tabs/day
Week 5: 400 mg injection, 5 tabs/day
Week 6: 300 mg injection, 4 tabs/day
Week 7: 200 mg injection, 3 tabs/day
Week 8: 100 mg injection, 2 tabs/day
Week 9: 2500 i.u. HCG/week
Week 10: 2500 i.u. HCG/week

THE ALLEGED LAST CYCLE USED BY THE LATE AUSTRIAN BODYBUILDER, ANDREAS MUNZER

Pro bodybuilder, Andreas Munzer died after having followed an extremely heavy cycle of drugs. There was no autopsy done, but rumor has it that his blood became very thick, he refused a transfusion, hemorrhaged into his stomach, and then died. From this description, it sounds like he died of complications resulting from diuretic use. As dehydration can lead to reduced blood volume and circulatory collapse. Aldactone is a diuretic that can cause gastric bleeding. Of course, given the volume of drugs he is known to have consumed (and chances are additional drugs we don't know about), the exact cause of his death will never be known.

The following is what is believed to be his drug use prior to his death:

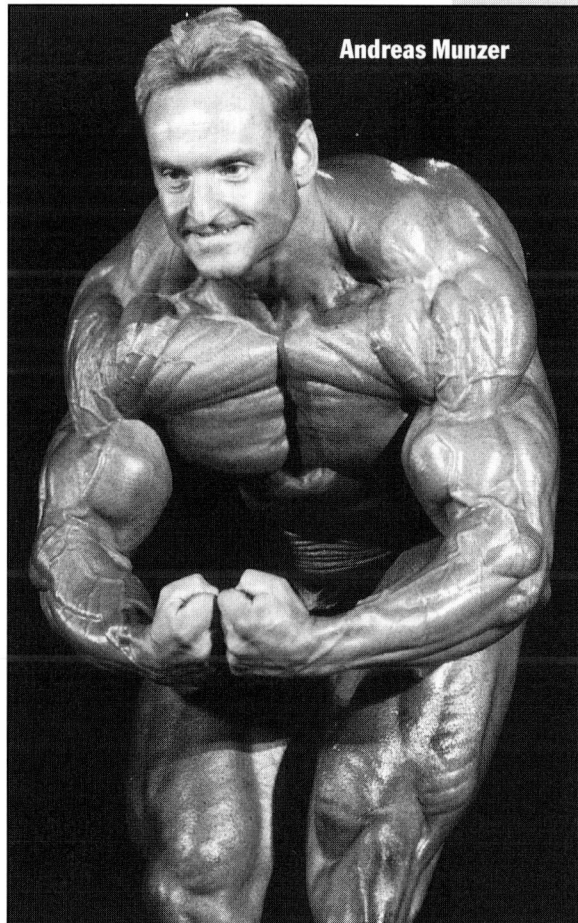

Andreas Munzer

All drugs listed were taken daily.

> 10 to 1 week prior to competition ptc: Thyroid Hormone
> 10 to 6 weeks ptc: Aspirin, Captagon, Clenbuterol, Ephedrine, AN1, Valium
> 8 to 6 weeks ptc: Testoviron 250 mg i.m., 2 times daily, Parabolan i.m , once a day, Halotestin 30 tablets, GH 24 i.e., Stromba i.m., 2 times daily, Stromba 50 tablets
> 5 to 3 weeks ptc: GH 24 i.e., Halotestin 30 tablets, Masteron i.m., 3 times daily, Parabolan i.m., 2 times daily , Stromba i.m., 2 times daily, Stromba 50 tablets
> 2 to 1 weeks ptc: GH 24 i.e., Halotestin 40 tablets, IGF-1, Insulin, Masteron i.m., 2 times a day, Stromba i.m., 2 times a day, Stromba 80 tablets
> Few days ptc: Aldactone, Lasix

If the previous is accurate, or even close to what most other pro bodybuilders are using, then we are surprised that more of them don't go the way of Munzer. A couple of cycles of one or two steroids is one thing, but the previous is polypharmacolgy at its worst. No one, and we mean NO ONE, knows what such drug combinations are doing to the human body. In Munzer's case they almost certainly led to his death. Unless there's a determined effort to clean up professional bodybuilding, we will probably see more pros heading to the great squat rack in the sky.

References
1) Physical-excellence@mail.com, Canada, *Musclenet Drus/Steroids Forum*, http://www.musclenet.com/steroid.htm.
2) marq@zen.co.uk, Subject: Save My Nuts, *Musclenet Drus/Steroids Forum*. http://www.musclenet.com/steroid.htm.
3) Cycle Theories, *Absolute Truth Hardcore Bodybuilding*,
☐ http://members.tripod.com/newgurus/cycletheories.htm.
4) David's Steroid Page, http:www.davids-steroidpage.com/.
5) Synovex, Drugs, *Absolute Truth Hardcore Bodybuilding*, http://www.geocities.com/HotSprings/2369/newsynovex.htm.
6) Finaplix, Drugs, *Absolute Truth Hardcore Bodybuilding*, http://www.geocities.com/HotSprings/2369/newfinaplix.htm.
7) Equipoise, Drugs, *Absolute Truth Hardcore Bodybuilding*, http://members.tripod.com/~newguru/newequipoise.html.
8) Primotestin Depot, Drugs, *Absolute Truth Hardcore Bodybuilding*, http://members.tripod.com/~newguru/newprimotestondepot.html.
9) Proviron, Drugs, *Absolute Truth Hardcore Bodybuilding*, http://www.geocities.com/HotSprings/2369/newproviron.htm.
10) Parabolan, Drugs, *Absolute Truth Hardcore Bodybuilding*, http://members.tripod.com/~newguru/newparabolan.html.
11) Masteron, Drugs, *Absolute Truth Hardcore Bodybuilding*, http://www.geocities.com/HotSprings/2369/newmasteron.htm.
12 Laurabolin, Drugs, *Absolute Truth Hardcore Bodybuilding*, http://members.tripod.com/~newguru/newlaurabolin.html.
13) Primobolan Depot, Drugs, *Absolute Truth Hardcore Bodybuilding*, http://members.tripod.com/~newguru/newprimobolandepot.html.
14) Winstrol, Drugs, *Absolute Truth Hardcore Bodybuilding*, http://members.tripod.com/~newguru/newwinstrol.html.
15) Durabolan, Drugs, *Absolute Truth Hardcore Bodybuilding*, http://members.tripod.com/~newguru/newdurabolon.html.
16) Dianabol, Drugs, *Absolute Truth Hardcore Bodybuilding*, http://members.tripod.com/~newguru/newdianabol.html.
17) Anavar, Drugs, *Absolute Truth Hardcore Bodybuilding*, http://members.tripod.com/~newguru/newanavar.html.
18) M,☐http://cpt.pixza/roids/M.htm.
19) I Had to Jab again, ☐http://www.anabolicsteroids.com/jabber.html.
20) Hormones and Synthetic substitutes, ☐http://heml.passagen.se/daho1000/may1997.html.
21) Hulkster's Newsletter,☐☐www.dclink.com/jaynik/april97.htm.
22) My first cycle, ☐www.dclink.com/jaynik/jun97.htm.

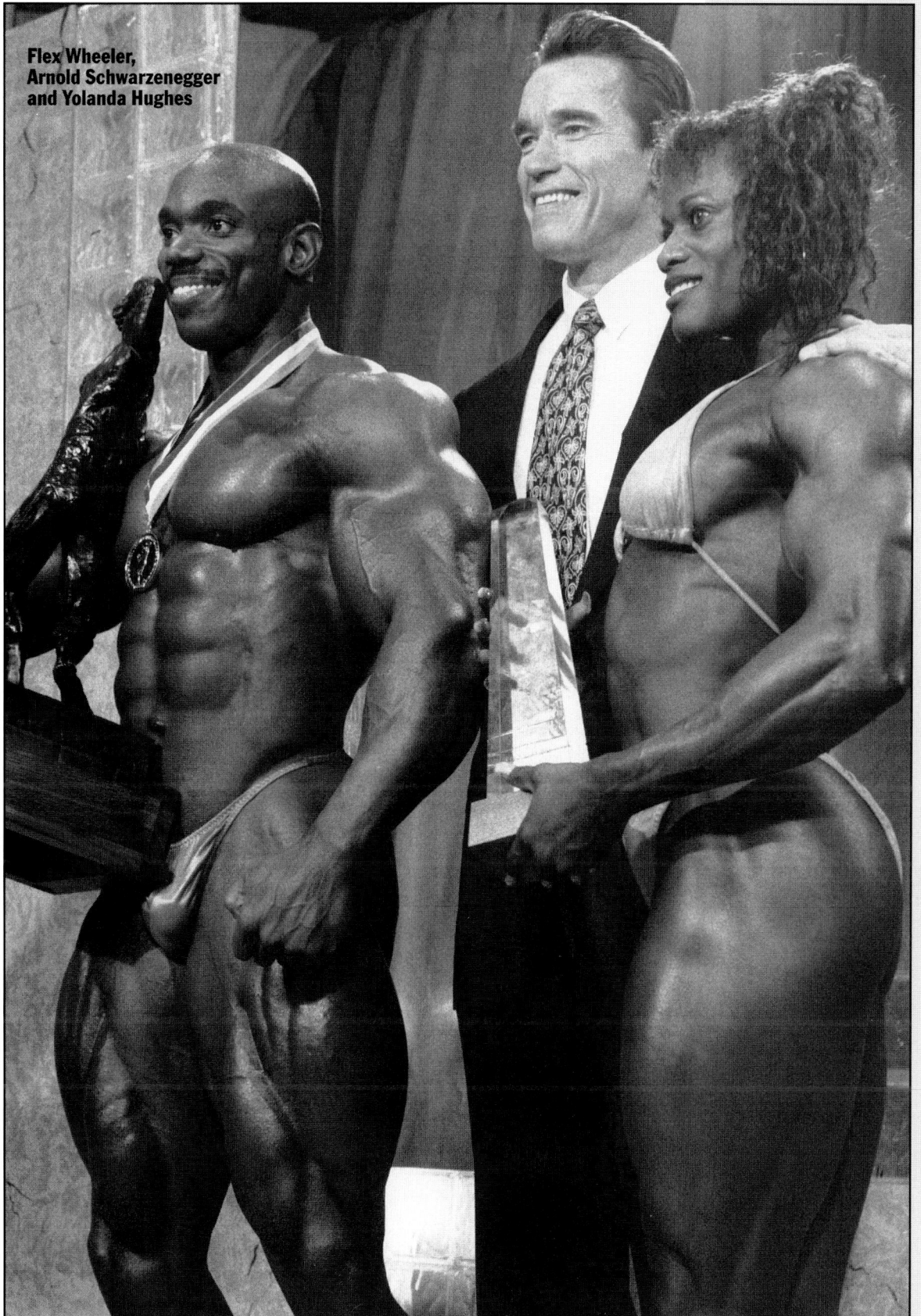

Flex Wheeler,
Arnold Schwarzenegger
and Yolanda Hughes

Glossary

Adaptogen – any substance that aids the body in fighting such internal and external stressers as the environment, pathogens and exercise.

Adrenaline – hormone released by the adrenal glands located on top of the kidneys. Adrenaline stimulates the sympathetic nervous system producing the "flight or fight" syndrome.

Agonist – substance that causes a desired response after stimulation of a given receptor system.

Aldosterone – body's primary water conserving hormone. Aldosterone works by stimulating the tubule cells of the kidney's to reabsorb minerals and water.

Amino acids – complex molecules composed of a central carbon atom, with an amine (NH3) group on one end and an acid (COOH) group on the other. Amino acids are often called the building blocks of life, and form polypeptide chains which in turn link together to form protein strands.

Anabolic steroids – group of substances designed to mimic the anabolic properties of testosterone, while minimizing the hormone's androgenic effects.

Antagonist – substance that acts opposite to an agonist, in that it prevents action at a given receptor system.

Antibiotic Growth Effect (AGE) – the increase in bodyweight that accompanies antibiotic administration in farm livestock.

Beta agonists – class of drugs that stimulate beta-receptors in the human body. Drugs that stimulate such receptors are primarily used for fat loss.

Biofeedback – process by which the body monitors and adjusts the level of circulating hormones.

Blood doping – general term used to describe any technique that increases the oxygen carrying capacity of the blood.

Desensitization – the diminished effect of a drug due to continued exposure.

Diuretics – any substance that speeds water excretion from the human body. Diuretics can be both synthetic drugs or natural (herbs).

Down regulation – decreased effect of a drug due to a decreased density of drug receptors.

Ecdysteroids – group of substances that produce molting in insects and crustaceans. In higher animals ecdysteroids produce an anabolic effect.

Electrolytes – electrically charged atoms (ions) that modify various body functions including heart rate, nervous conduction and water retention.

Enzyme – peptide based substance that helps regulate biochemical reactions. Enzymes don't start reactions, but speed existing ones.

Erythropoietin (EPO) – hormone released by the kidneys that increases red blood cell production. EPO is one of the primary methods of blood doping.

Estrogen – sex hormone that produces feminizing effects and plays a major role in the female reproductive system. Both men's and women's bodies contain estrogen, but because it is found in much higher concentrations in women's bodies, the hormone is often called "a female hormone."

Glycogen – the stored form of sugar. It is primarily found in the liver and skeletal muscles.

Gym dosage – amount of a drug taken by athletes to boost athletic performance or increase muscle size and strength. In most cases the gym dosage is far above the therapeutic dosage.

Herb – any plant or shrub that is taken for medical purposes. Herbs form the nucleus of alternative forms of medicine.

Hormone – peptide (protein) or steroid based substance that modifies or stimulates various metabolic pathways.

Hyperglycemia – term used to indicate high blood sugar levels.

Hypoglycemia – term used to describe low blood sugar levels.

Insulin – body's primary nutrient storage hormone. Insulin is produced by the pancreas and controls the level of such substances as glucose and amino acids.

Lipogenesis – the process by which the body manufactures new fat molecules from precursor molecules.

Lipolysis – process by which triglycerides are broken down into glycerol, and fatty acids are broken down into acetyl-COA and then fed into the citric acid cycle to produce ATP.

Narcotic analgesics – group of substances derived from opium alkaloids, that are primarily used to kill pain.

Neurotransmitter – any substance that is used to relay messages within the brain.

Peptide – another name for amino acid. Peptide chains are strings of amino acids linked together by high energy bonds.

Permeability – the property that describes a membrane's ability to absorb fluids and dissolved substances.

Ph scale – measure of the amount of H+ and OH- ions in solution. The Ph scale ranges from one to 14 with one representing most acid (highest concentration of H+ ions) and 14 representing most basic (highest concentration of OH- ions).

Prostaglandins – hormone-like substances made from fatty acids that are involved in such processes as protein synthesis, blood pressure regulation and digestion.

Protein – collection of peptide (amino acids) chains that serves as the building material for most of the human body.

Receptor – site on or within a cell that interacts with a given substance (usually a drug) to produce a biological response. Most receptors are specific for one drug.

Stimulants – any substance that speeds up the central nervous system or one of its subsystems. The primary effects of stimulants are increased heart rate, increased respiratory rate and increased mental alertness.

Testosterone – sex hormone that produces both anabolic (muscle building) and androgenic (secondary sex characteristics) effects. Both men and women have testosterone in their bodies, but because of the much higher concentrations in men's bodies the hormone is often called "a male hormone."

Therapeutic dosage – the amount of a drug given for medical treatment.

Thermogenesis – process of fat oxidation, produced when an elevation of body temperature liberates fat stores.

Thyroid drugs – synthetic derivatives of the body's naturally occurring thyroid hormones T3, thyronine, and T4, thyroxine. Athletes use thyroid drugs to speed up the body's metabolism and increase fat oxidation.

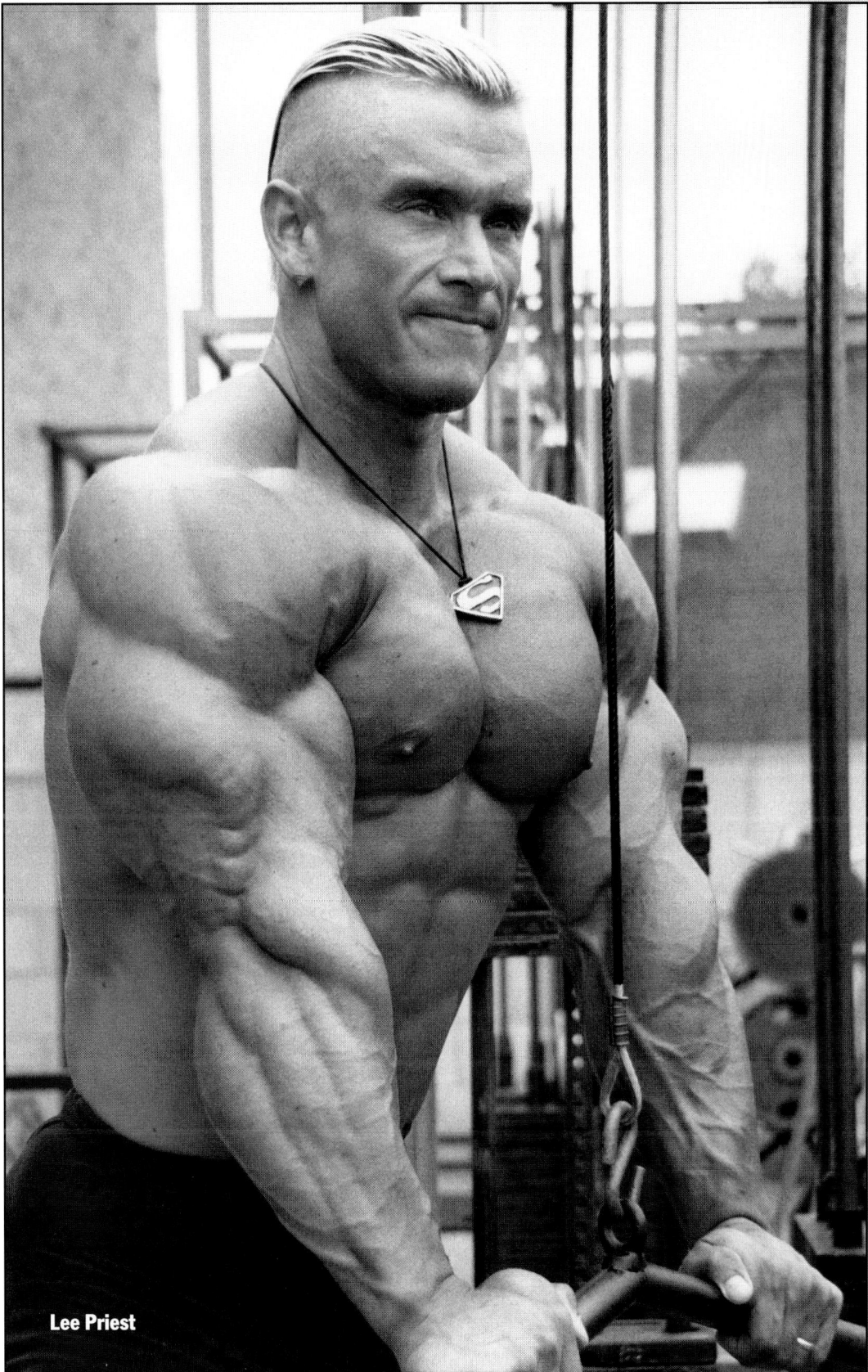

Lee Priest

INDEX

A

Acetazolamide, 92
Acetyl-L-carnitine (ACL), 72
    effects of, 72
Acne, 62
Adenosine triphosphate (ATP), 30
Adipocytes, 47
Adipose tissue, 44
AGE (antibiotic growth effect), 52, 53
Aging, 69
Aggressiveness, 16, 62
Agrimony (agrimonia eupatoria), 91
    dosage, 91
AIDS, 95
Aladiene, 92
Alanine, 74
Alatone (spironolactone), 93
Aldactone (spironolactone), 89, 92, 93
    dosage of, 89
    effects of, 89
Aldosterone, 83, 84
Aldosterone antagonists, 89
    effect of, 89
    example of, 89
Amaryl (glimepiride), 110
    dosage of, 110
    effects of, 110
Amiloride, 92
Amphetamines, 103
    examples of, 103-105
Anabolic steroids, 14-29, 53, 66
    legality of, 14
    side effects of, 14
    teenagers and, 14
Anadiol (testosterone suspension), 23
    dosage of, 23
    effects of, 23
Anadrol (oxymetholone), 15
    dosage of, 15
    effects of, 15
Anadrol 50 (oxymetholone), 15
    dosage of, 15
    effects of, 15
Analgesia, 39
Anapolon 50 (oxymetholone), 15
    dosage of, 15
    effects of, 15
Anasteron (oxymetholone), 15
    dosage of, 15
    effects of, 15
Anatest (testosterone suspension), 23
    dosage of, 23
    effects of, 23
Anavar (oxandrolone), 21
    dosage of, 21
    effects of, 21
Andriol (testosterone undecanoate), 15
    dosage of, 15
    effects of, 15
Android (methyltestosterone), 21
    dosage of, 21
    effects of, 21
Android-F (fluoxymesterone), 16
    dosage of, 16, 63
    effects of, 16
    side effects of, 16
Androstenedione, 58, 60-63, 64, 67
    effects of, 61-62
    side effects of, 62
Androtardyl (testosterone enanthate), 23
    dosage of, 23
    effects of, 23
Androxen (testosterone undecanoate), 15
    dosage of, 15
    effects of, 15
Androyd (oxymetholone), 15
    dosage of, 15
    effects of, 15
Anemia, 94, 95
Anhydron (cyclothiazide), 88
    dosage of, 88
Antibiotics as growth promotants, 52-53
    bodybuilding applications, 53
    effects of, 52-53
    examples of, 53
    negative effects of, 53
Anticatabolic, 66
Antidiuretic hormone (ADH), 83
Antihyperglycemic, 108

Antitriol (oxandrolone), 21
    dosage of, 21
    effects of, 21
Aphrodisiac, 70
Aquatag (benzthiazide), 88, 92
    dosage of, 88
Ardomon (clomiphene citrate), 25-26
    dosage of, 25
    effects of, 26
    side effects of, 26
Arnold, Patrick, 67
Aromatization, 66
Arthritis, 69
Atom, 59
ATP-citrate lyase, 51
Autologous, 94
Autonomic nervous system (ANS), 79

B

Bacitracin, 53
Bacteria, 52
Bambermycins, 53
Bearberry (arctostaphylos uva-ursi), 91
    dosage of, 91
Bendroflumethiazide, 92
Benzothiadiazides (thiazides), 87-88
    effects of, 87
    examples of, 88
    side effects of, 87-88
    therapeutic use of, 88
Benzthiamide, 92
Bergmottin, 32
Beta agonists, 44-48
    effects of, 45-46
    effects on prostaglandins, 46
    examples of, 45-46
Beta receptors, 44
    down-regulation and desensitization, 47
    subtypes of, 44
        beta-1, 44
        beta-2, 44, 45, 47
        beta-3, 44, 45, 47-48
            benefits of, 48
            examples of, 48
            side effects of, 47-48
            studies of, 47
Biguanides, 108
    examples of, 108-111
Biofeedback, 116
Bioflavonoids, 69
Birth control pills, 68
Blood, 94-99
Blood buffering, 97-98
    biochemistry of, 97
    human applications, 97
    sodium bicarbonate (NaHCO₃), 98
Blood doping, 94-95
    how it's done, 94-95
        Epogen, 95
        Epoetin, 95-96
            testing for, 96
Blood transfusion, 94
Blue flag (iris versicolor), 91
    dosage of, 91
Boldebol-H (boldenone undecylenate), 18
    dosage of, 18
    effects of, 18
Boldenone 50 (boldenone undecylenate), 18
    dosage of, 18
    effects of, 18
Boldenone undecylenate, 18
    dosage of, 18
    effects of, 18
Boldo (peumus boldo), 91
    dosage of, 91
Bone marrow, 96
Boneset (eupatorium perfoliatum), 91
    dosage of, 91
Boxers, 21
Breast cancer, 27
Broom (sarothamnus scoparius), 91
    dosage of, 91
Buchu (barosma betulina), 91
    dosage of, 91
Buffering agents, 94
Bugleweed (lycopus europaeus), 91
    dosage of, 91
Bumetanide, 90
    dosage of, 90
    side effects of, 90

Contributing Photographers
Josef Adlt, Jim Amentler, Angelo Bani, Skip Faulkner,
Irvin Gelb, Robert Kennedy, Ricky Marconi,
Jason Mathas, Mitsuru Okabe, David Paul, Ove Rytter,
Dennis Warren, Art Zeller